"Ginny Mills and her staff are extremely caring and helpful. They know what it is like to feel lost, scared, and not know where to turn for help for addiction. They look at each situation, what the immediate needs are, and develop a plan.... Ginny helped save my family and gave us hope again."

—Trish S., North Carolina

"The knowledge we gained on how to deal with our son's addiction during our meetings with Ginny was and remains irreplaceable. Ginny listened to us and helped us to communicate love, compassion and boundaries with our son. She made sure we took care of ourselves. She helped us reach the point where we were able to trust the process. Ginny is so professional, passionate, knowledgeable, calm and truly terrific. "

—Doug R., New York

"Because of our work with Ginny, we went from lacking confidence and feeling confused and afraid to feeling much more calm, confident and well-equipped to respond to our son along his recovery journey, no matter what twists and turns could lie ahead. "

—Suzanne F., Georgia

"Ginny Mills provided our family with an incredible amount of compassion, support and professionalism. S' ·ided us with clear guidance b   edge and experience. Ginny wa   and it turned out to be one o   ver made. It is a journey, but   1ow have hope."

—Larry O., North Carolina

"When our son was struggling with addiction we did not realize the best way to help him was by helping ourselves. Through Parenting Through Addiction and Ginny Mills we were able to learn more about addiction as well as specific ways to handle certain situations and talk to our child. Especially important was learning how to do things together as a team."

—Glenn and Suzanne F., Georgia

"Working with Ginny was one of the most helpful parts of our recovery experience as a family. We have had many counselors throughout the years and Ginny, by far, has been the most helpful to us, as parents. It is so helpful to know that we can continue working with Ginny even as our son transitions from one program to another."

—Jeff C., Tennessee

"My first contact with Ginny was pure serendipity... When she returned my call, she literally changed our lives. I was terrified and at a total loss for how to help without good information. Ginny was able to educate me, define appropriate options, explain the disease and offer hope, all while helping me learn how to talk to my daughter and our other family members. The learning curve is steep and the lack of information and maze of options is daunting. No one can navigate this life-changing tragedy without support. Ginny's voice of hope and compassion led us out of the chaos and to a path of sustainable sobriety.

—Carolyn M., North Carolina

"Ginny Mills has helped me as a pastor understand practical aspects of helping families who struggle with addiction. Her insights on how to encourage parents, while providing solid guidance to individuals in addiction, has been a strong resource in my ministry. I am very grateful for her new book: Parenting Through Your Adult Child's Addiction. It has become the most practical resource to share with others struggling through the journey of addiction. It provides keen insight along with practical steps. She offers information specific to parents as well as individuals working to overcome addiction. The best aspect of this resource is how it helps pastors (or other non-licensed counselors) to grasp the uniqueness of the journey of addiction intervention and recovery for both the individual working through an addiction and their family and friends."

—*Rev. Dr. Neil Routh*
Grace Moravian Church, Mount Airy, NC

PARENTING THROUGH YOUR ADULT CHILD'S ADDICTION

Making Sense of Treatment, Aftercare, and Recovery Recommendations

GINNY H. MILLS
Family Recovery Specialist
MAED, LCAS, LPCS

CONTENTS

Introduction 1

1 | How Did We Get Here? 3

2 | Getting Help and Following Initial
Recommendations 19

3 | Residential Treatment is Like the Classroom
Part of Driver's Ed 37

4 | Learning in the Classroom and Preparing for
the Road 53

5 | Profiles to Illustrate 81

6 | Parent Profiles 93

7 | Support for Families 115

8 | In Conclusion 119

INTRODUCTION

No parent imagines that their tiny baby, kindergartener, ballerina, or Pop Warner running back will one day grow up to have an addiction. No one. It seems impossible that our once precious child grew up to make such frightening choices and take such terrifying risks. Yet here you are, trying to learn what you can do as a family member without revealing the resentments, doubts, fears, and expectations you harbor.

Recognizing the need for a recovery program, finding a way to pay for it, and getting your child through the door can be overwhelming enough.

If the treatment journey has begun, the staff may be talking about him having a "disease," like somehow that justifies the lies, manipulation, sleepless nights, and awful things he has said and done. The staff says that "she's sick, not bad."

When you hear the word "sick," it is tempting to compare addiction recovery to recovery from other acute illnesses like appendicitis or a broken ankle. Most parents can relate to that kind of recovery, but most have not witnessed addiction recovery. Instead, this book offers a comparison to something almost *every parent* can relate to – *their child learning how to drive.*

To that end, each chapter ends with a Driving Lesson for an Adult Child with Addiction and one for Parents.

Some of us read every word of parenting guides, newspaper articles, and user agreements. Others seem to get the key points and move on. Regardless of which kind of reader you are, we hope that the combination of full chapters and "Driving Lessons" will be helpful.

 "Driving Lessons for an Adult Child with Addiction" are offered to give you—the parent—language to convey key information to your son or daughter. They may not entirely grasp or agree, but at least you'll have some brief statements to use as words of encouragement. Remember, brief statements work better than long lectures or extensive pleading. Make your point and encourage them to consider it, then let it go and see what happens.

 "Driving Lessons for Parents" are offered to help you grasp the most important information from that chapter as well. If you remember nothing else, we hope you'll hold onto those key points. You can download a copy of the Driving Lessons from our resource page for the book at:

www.parentingthroughaddiction.com/TheBook

CHAPTER ONE

HOW DID WE GET HERE?

By now, it is likely that you are worried your son or daughter's use of drugs or alcohol has reached a sufficient level of concern that you are exploring or have already admitted your son or daughter to treatment.

That means you've already been through a lot. You've ranted and punished, cried and pleaded, and it may have felt like nothing seemed to matter. You knew your child would one day become a teenager and throw you new curveballs, but you had hoped to avoid this one. Yet here you are.

Using alcohol or even some drugs, along with sexual behavior, are considered "adult activities" and thus often perceived by teens as "rites of passage," just like being able to drive.

In most states, students are eligible for enrollment in driver's education by age fifteen. When we think about our own teenage years, we may remember feeling grown up or terrified when it was our time to start learning to drive. But when your own teen was ready to sign up for driver's ed, you probably weren't ready at all! After all, this was the same kid who, just a few years ago, laughed uproariously at bathroom humor or was agonizing over being old enough to get her ears pierced!

The scary part is that, just as our teens were learning to demonstrate abstract thought and pay more attention to the world around them (skills they need for learning how to drive), they were also exposed to opportunities to experiment with alcohol or other drugs. They experimented because they were curious – or they wanted to fit in – or both. Soon though, some people find both reward *and* relief in the use of alcohol or other drugs. What started as a typical adolescent experiment began to take on a life of its own. For some, that developed into full-blown addiction.

It is pretty overwhelming to realize that your child – the same kid you took to summer camp and who performed beautifully in the dance recital, gymnastics meet, soccer match, or science fair competition – has behaved their way into getting sick. Really sick.

Here's the way the progression usually goes:

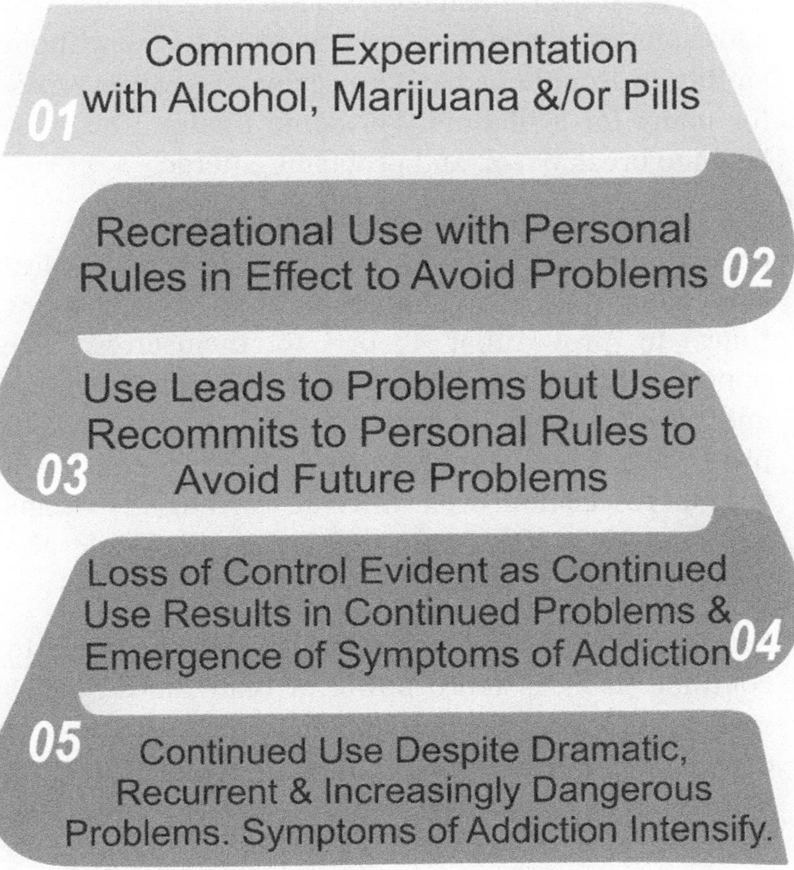

01 Common Experimentation with Alcohol, Marijuana &/or Pills

Recreational Use with Personal Rules in Effect to Avoid Problems **02**

03 Use Leads to Problems but User Recommits to Personal Rules to Avoid Future Problems

Loss of Control Evident as Continued Use Results in Continued Problems & Emergence of Symptoms of Addiction **04**

05 Continued Use Despite Dramatic, Recurrent & Increasingly Dangerous Problems. Symptoms of Addiction Intensify.

Figure 1: Progression from Experimentation to Addiction

Stage 1: Experimentation, unless it resulted in a bad experience, typically leads to the desire to use again.

Stage 2: Non-Problematic Use. Recreational use with conscious or unconscious rules in place to use without getting in trouble or having problems – which works for many for a lifetime. For some though, the rules begin to break down, and problems emerge.

The movement from Stage 2 to Stage 3 is where the opportunity for learning exists. "If x, then y." Typical adolescents need to conduct that experiment a few times to prove that theory to themselves. The opportunity can be helpful for many, as long as parents and others do not prevent learning by rescuing and protecting from consequences. For others, even without rescue (and even with true learning), problems will continue because the user is losing control, despite best intentions.

Stage 3: When problems start to happen, the desire to continue using is more powerful than the desire to stop, and as long as there has not yet been a loss of control, the individual recommits to personal rules and thus avoids having more problems in the future. This means making a sincere and committed attempt to return to Stage 2. For individuals whose use has not progressed to the point that they have lost control, this effort can actually be successful.

The movement from Stage 3 to Stage 4 can best be categorized as the point at which control is lost. This can be characterized as "the point of no return." It is like an unmarked border crossing in the snow, in the fog and in the dark. If people knew where it was, they would never cross it, and they don't realize they've crossed it when they do.

This line is "the point of no return."

Stage 4: For some though, that attempt to reclaim the Stage 2 status just doesn't work because their ability to control the outcome is just not there. Notice the keyword *ability*, not *willingness*. The willingness could be there, but the ability is lost. By this point, continued use will undoubtedly lead to continued problems and the emergence of further symptoms of addiction.

Stage 5: By the time users reach this stage, there really seems to be no question that a pattern has emerged. Typically, some periods seem to be less chaotic than others, but in general, symptoms of true addiction are unmistakable. Crises create pain points for parents to offer treatment, but depending on the readiness of the user, acceptance of treatment may or may not require repeated crises and pain points.

Where Do We Go from Here?

In reflecting on your son or daughter's patterns of use, you may feel confidence that there is reason for alarm and a strong need for your adult child to get help to stop the progression before it gets any worse. However, your readiness for your adult child to make change and theirs may differ.

DiClemente, Prochaska, Miller and others identified distinctive stages of change for all of us, not just those affected by substance use disorders. Learning how to recognize those stages of change can help parents better understand that willingness to make change is correlated with the awareness of a need to change. Many people simply do not recognize the need until they gain enough information.

An Overview of the Stages of Change:

- **Pre-contemplation** – lack of awareness of need to change, therefore no motivation to do so. With substance use, this stage is characterized by frustration demonstrated by the person who is being encouraged to make change (largely because they see the change as unnecessary and undesirable).

- **Contemplation** – increased awareness about a possible need to change but ambivalence based on positive reasons to continue a current behavior. Although encouraging, this stage is characterized primarily by thinking about making change without a decision to do so.

- **Preparation** – increased awareness and acceptance of a need to change, but perhaps with regret that change is necessary. This stage is characterized by the decision to make change but often with ongoing hope that such change might not have to happen.

- **Action** – awareness, acceptance, decision and intentional efforts to make change. This stage is characterized by genuine effort to make change, but not necessarily with enthusiasm, conviction or delight.

- **Maintenance** – deliberate efforts to sustain changes already made. This stage is characterized by an increased ease to sustain the changes and often with appreciation that the change is positive for one's self.

- **Regression** (or relapse) – the individual returns to behaviors that have previously been changed. This stage is characterized by a return to old thoughts, perceptions, or feelings that allowed ambivalence to return.

Parents may sense that there is a problem with substance use long before their son or daughter. There can be value in understanding that the person who is pre-contemplative simply lacks adequate information to conclude that change is needed.

Of course, there are some benefits to not making change, such as the opportunity to continue using alcohol or other drugs, with or without the goal of experiencing intoxication or impairment. Contemplating or reflecting on those benefits contributes to ambivalence about making change.

Recognizing where your son or daughter is in the change process can help you appreciate how close or how far they may be from being ready to consider intentional change.

Ironically, an individual can reach the Action Stage of change and become ready to make intentional change, but those changes may not be as broad in scope as a parent might want. For example, your daughter may experience great distress following an alcohol-induced blackout and decide that she is not going to drink alcohol again. But since blackouts are not experienced with marijuana use, she may plan to continue marijuana use, much to your dismay. Such change is meaningful and can be quite genuine, but you may have a strong desire for her to become willing to choose recovery and abstinence from all substances, not just abstinence from alcohol.

That could simply mean that your daughter lacks the awareness and understanding that, for those with the disease of addiction, any continued use of controlled substances is likely to continue creating pain and unmanageability in her life.

When parents enable, rescue, or otherwise interfere with the opportunity for their son or daughter to gain the information, insight, or awareness of the ways in which substance use is negatively affecting their lives, parents slow down the progression through the stages of change. Unfortunately, with the disease of addiction, that information usually comes in the form of distress.

Ideally, your son or daughter can admit to treatment in the preparation or action stage of change in order to get the most benefit from treatment.

Sometimes though, the "fog" of the delusional belief that everything is really okay despite very serious addictions, such as heroin, crack cocaine, meth-amphetamine or IV drug use, warrants admission to treatment as soon as possible, even if they have not yet experienced a moment of clarity that helps them begin contemplating change. It may require a period of enforced abstinence for the "fog" to lift so they can reflect on the reality of their life.

THE POWER OF PAIN

Pain creates moments of clarity, and when an offer for an alternative form of relief intersects with a moment of clarity, that is when the crisis becomes a perfect opportunity.

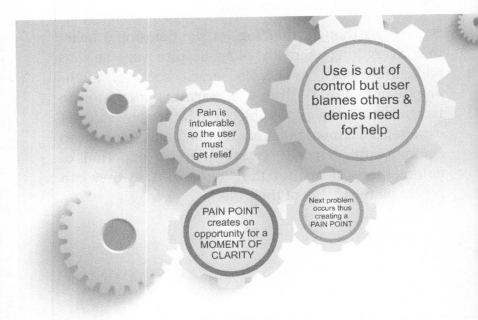

Figure 2: Pain leads to clarity & opportunity

No parent truly wants their son or daughter to hurt, but in truth, those pain points are opportunities. If you miss one, if your son or daughter's use of substances has progressed to addiction, don't worry, you'll unfortunately have another opportunity. Each crisis is an opportunity to invite your son or daughter with addiction to accept help and begin recovery.

Often though, the denial and delay tactics of the pre-contemplative through the preparation stages of change result in their determination to hold out as long as possible. The notion of "I've still got time" often results in delaying or stalling until the pain is simply unbearable. That pain can lead to "the gift of desperation," and that gift can lead to a new willingness to ask for and/or accept help when they had rejected it before.

Parents can *help that moment come sooner* by fighting the temptation to offer rescue from responsibilities, consequences, and financial or legal problems. It is especially important that parents avoid helping them continue to use drugs or alcohol.

Addiction treatment – either residential or intensive outpatient – is an appropriate resource when substance use has progressed to addiction, but sometimes it is hard to know if there's enough evidence to support such a diagnosis. Although numerous elements help independent addiction specialists determine the severity of the drug or alcohol problem, the official diagnosis is perhaps most relevant.

IS IT REALLY ADDICTION?

By the time your son or daughter needs treatment, four or more of the following symptoms of addiction should be evident:

- Using more of the substance or using it for longer than really intended, aka "Loss of Control." *Yeah, I didn't mean to blackout, but hey, it happens. Actually, it happens a lot.*

- Time spent seeking, using, and recovering from using the drug is extensive. *It gets almost all my attention.*

- Craving and preoccupation. *It's all I can think about. Sometimes I even feel it in my body.*

- Unsuccessful efforts to quit or cut down. *I can quit. I just don't stay quit.*

- Repeatedly unable to meet responsibilities at school, home, or work because of using. *Yeah, I really don't care that much about school now. I used to think I'd go to college, but that's probably not going to happen.*

- Stopping or reducing important social, occupational, or recreational activities. *That thing I used to love doing more than life itself? Yeah, I don't do that anymore.*

- Continued use despite persistent or recurring social or relationship problems caused by using.

The biggest problem I have with my using is that my parents just will not let up! We fight about it all the time, but that's not going to stop me from doing my favorite thing.

- Repeated use in dangerous situations. *I love to get stoned, go driving, really crank up my music, and just ride.*

- Continued use even though using causes or makes worse a physical or psychological problem. *I know that getting high interferes with my meds, but I really don't care. I don't think they work anyway! But getting high makes me feel better every single time!*

- It takes more and more of the substance – or a shift to a more potent substance – to achieve the desired results. *Yeah, it just didn't do it for me anymore. That's why I switched to _____.*

- If the use of the substance is stopped, characteristic withdrawal symptoms occur; or the substance is used specifically to avoid experiencing withdrawal symptoms. *I don't really even use drugs to get high anymore. I just don't want to get dope sick.*

For a worksheet on applying what you have learned about symptoms, visit:

www.parentingthroughaddiction.com/ TheBook

The Truth about Detox

Withdrawal symptoms from cocaine, methamphetamine, LSD, MDMA (Ecstasy & Molly), and marijuana are evident but not dangerous. Heroin and opiate withdrawal is miserable but not dangerous. The most dangerous withdrawal or detox is from alcohol and benzodiazepines (like the more common drugs Xanax (alprazolam), Klonopin (clonazepam), Ativan (lorazepam), or Valium (diazepam) as well as less commonly known drugs like etizolam. Even teens and young adults may need a medically-monitored detox if their primary use has been heavy daily alcohol or benzodiazepine.

In most cases, teens and young adults have limited need for medically monitored detox, but those whose use of opiates or heroin has been significant can benefit from medication and support in a clinical setting, primarily for comfort.

It can take as long as six weeks for the body to excrete all the THC from heavy marijuana smokers (especially those who use butane hash oil, cannabis oil, "wax," "shatter," "dabs" or strains of marijuana that have exceptionally high levels of THC).

Striking while the Iron is Hot

Take a moment to reflect back on Figure 2, the Pain Point graphic. If you were fortunate enough to secure admission to treatment for your son or daughter in that moment of clarity, there's a good chance your child moved from the Contemplation to the Action Stage of Change. If that hasn't happened yet, then now is the time to do the following:

- Actively start learning everything you can about addiction and recovery.

- Find your tribe of parents who are struggling with the same challenges. It won't make it easy, but it will help to find other parents who "get it."

- Identify an independent addiction specialist to help you learn about treatment resources and get help for yourself.

- Choose at least one treatment program that seems to be a good fit for your family's needs, preferences, and resources.

- Reduce your enabling behaviors and wait for a crisis.

- When the crisis occurs, recognize the opportunity and extend the offer for treatment.

When a parent makes the decision to reach out to a professional for help, whether it is for your son or daughter or for yourself, the recovery journey has begun.

Driving Lessons

 For an Adult Child with Addiction: Establishing recovery is easier when there is less wreckage and less progression of the disease.

 For Parents: Even if your son or daughter isn't "action ready," that doesn't mean there is nothing you can do. Conventional wisdom has told you to "wait until they hit bottom and go to Al-Anon." New wisdom acknowledges that there can be many opportunities (or many "bottoms") that can create willingness to accept help. In anticipation of willingness, there are many things you can do because you are action-ready.

Chapter Two

Getting Help and Following Initial Recommendations

With the decision to reach out to a professional for help, that independent addiction specialist likely recommended that your son or daughter "get some driving lessons" because the recovery journey is not one to be embarked upon alone. Rarely does the bootstrapping method work when it comes to this disease.

"Wait, what?" you say. "Who said anything about a disease?" Well, once that shift from Stage 3 to Stage 4 happens, there's a pretty good chance that your son or daughter has the disease of addiction.

And "what's wrong with bootstrapping?! I mean seriously! If he would get a job and start acting like an adult instead of a lazy bum, this thing would take care of itself." The bootstrapping approach, when applied to addiction, is the equivalent of saying to your son with a brain tumor, "You just need to get yourself together and stop complaining! We all have headaches sometimes, and we just have to push through it. We have and so will you!"

THE DISEASE CONCEPT IS NOT NEW NEWS

The American Medical Association first recognized addiction as a disease in 1956.[1] Then in 2011, the American Society of Addiction Medicine offered a much more specific description of addiction as a brain disease, not simply a behavioral problem associated with using drugs, alcohol, gambling, or sex.

> "At its core, addiction isn't just a social problem or a moral problem or a criminal problem. It's a brain problem whose behaviors manifest in all these other areas," said Dr. Michael Miller, past president of ASAM who oversaw the development of the new definition. "Many behaviors driven by addiction are real problems and sometimes criminal acts. But the disease is about brains, not drugs. It's about underlying neurology, not outward actions."

Long before that, a 1938 report from the Scientific Committee of the Research Council on Problems of Alcohol Commission[2] stated that "an alcoholic should be regarded as a sick person, just as one who is suffering from tuberculosis, cancer, heart disease, or any other serious chronic condition." We can trace the

---

[1] https://www.asam.org/docs/pressreleases/asam-definition-of-addiction-2011-08-15.pdf
[2] Reports: The Research Council on Problems of Alcohol. *Science.* 1938a; 88:329–332.
https://science.sciencemag.org/content/88/2284/329.2

concept of alcoholism and addiction as a disease all the way back to Dr. Benjamin Rush (who also was one of the signers of the Constitution) who defined the disease process of alcoholism in 1784.[3]

In 1937, Dr. William Silkworth equated alcoholism with an allergy – a concept that is simple enough to understand, but also not diagnosable in the same way doctors diagnose other allergies. Nevertheless, the idea made so much sense that it led to Dr. Silkworth's contribution of the chapter entitled "The Doctor's Opinion" in the classic text, *Alcoholics Anonymous.*

For those who wish to read Dr. Silkworth's seminal work, follow the link below:

http://silkworth.net/gsowatch/litbook.pdf

In the previous chapter, one model of the stages of progression was briefly outlined, and the diagnostic conditions were explained. As hard as it may be to believe, if your son or daughter has progressed to Stage 4 and meets at least four of those diagnostic criteria, it is safe to say that a diagnosis of the disease of addiction is appropriate.

If Dr. Silkworth's description of addiction as an allergy or the AMA conclusions of over sixty years ago isn't convincing enough that addiction is a disease, you might appreciate hearing from a current thought

---

[3] Rush, Dr. Benjamin. *An Inquiry Into the Effects of Ardent Spirits on the Human Mind and Body*
https://www.smithsonianmag.com/smart-news/how-colonial-doctor-changed-medical-views-alcohol-180955813/#fLou3jSUIRBx2QWD.99

leader in the field. Dr. Kevin McCauley offers great insights in his video *Pleasure Unwoven.* Dr. McCauley shares his own journey of trying to understand how his own diagnosis of addiction eventually made sense for him as a physician. Dr. McCauley admits that he firmly rejected the disease argument when he was in treatment, but he became a believer based on his own independent research. You may want to check out his free video clips on YouTube by following this link:

https://youtu.be/wxiKVQR90VM

Dr. McCauley also addresses the Choice Theory in a separate section of the video.

https://youtu.be/u_scpXuE4rk

In that segment, he discusses the argument that addiction cannot be a disease because people choose to use alcohol or drugs. *Pleasure Unwoven* offers a helpful overview of understanding addiction as a disease, described by a medical doctor and former skeptic. You can purchase the whole video on Amazon or rent or buy it to stream through Vimeo On-Demand.

But Aren't There Exceptions?

It's true that addiction specialists must acknowledge that there really are those who look like they have addiction at one time in their life, never get treatment, then appear to be able to make changes with no treatment or recovery activities. Some men returned from Vietnam who used heroin there, yet did not use heroin on their return to the United States. There are those who abused drugs or drank heavily in college then grew up and moved on with their lives, leaving the party lifestyle behind as they accepted adult responsibilities.

Those people almost certainly met the definition of "heavy user" but were probably not truly sick with the disease of addiction. However, the odds are not good that your son or daughter is one of those exceptions. We would argue that it's preferable to take the "better safe than sorry" approach... aka, "Get recommendations from an independent addiction specialist and follow those recommendations just as you would with an oncologist."

We know that helping families understand addiction as it compares to other medical conditions is hard. It is so easy to want a quick fix or a "one and done" experience with getting treatment. Sometimes one very effective episode of treatment can work, especially when the patient is a highly-motivated person who knows they are sick.

For many others though, the journey to sustainable recovery is not nearly as linear. That, indeed, is the reason this book was written! We want to introduce you now to the reality that recovery is a long process that begins with the initial willingness to accept outside help, but it can be fraught with many pitfalls, twists, and turns... some of which can indeed be avoided!

We invite you to discover how you can be part of the solution:

- Continue to learn. There are a variety of resources available to help you begin to grasp what addiction is like for your adult child and what makes recovery so challenging.

- Stay engaged with your "tribe." Arrive early and hang around after meetings to chat and get phone numbers from other parents. Explore opportunities for getting together for dinner after a meeting or meeting for coffee. There is great value in connecting with other parents who understand the experience.

- Continue efforts to eliminate enabling your adult child's drug or alcohol use to continue. This means avoiding the temptation to rescue them from consequences, lie or cover up for them, pay for their mistakes by paying fines, fees, bail, etc., or do tasks for them that they can and should do for themselves. You might even want to seek coaching and accountability to eliminate as many enabling behaviors as you can.

- Discontinue all "spy game" activity. Even though you might tell yourself that you feel better knowing where your adult child is, how and where he or she is spending money, or whether they are bringing drugs in your home, it is like a worm hole in space! What began as responsible parental monitoring can become (and may already be) an obsessive-compulsive behavior. It doesn't accomplish anything anyway, so practice your own abstinence from that behavior. Consider the equivalent of asking your adult child to stop using drugs or alcohol.

- Stay in touch with your independent addiction specialist, education consultant, or care coordination group. You want to have all the information for one or two appropriate treatment program(s) so you are ready to take action in response to a crisis.

- Actively nurture your other relationships. If you are married or in a relationship, make date nights a priority again. If you have other children, make a point of spending time with them and talking about what's going on in their lives.

- Live your life! This could be a long journey, so you cannot afford to put your job, your own healthcare, your relationships, or even your vacation on hold forever. By now we hope you have accepted that you cannot control your adult child's behavior, so recommit to living your own life in a whole, healthy way at the same time you ask them to take responsibility for doing the same.

- Stay open to the many paths to recovery for your adult child while recognizing that, whichever path is chosen, it will likely take 5+ years to sustained remission.

Gaining Perspective about Treatment by Considering Other Conditions

Consider the differences between commonly diagnosed and treated conditions, based on the number of care visits, length of primary treatment and aftercare follow-up.

This comparison offers some valuable perspectives to help families know what to expect.

Condition: Strep Throat

Primary treatment: 1-2 visits to primary care physician and a full course of antibiotics

Recuperation after treatment: 4-5 days

Time to full recovery: 10 days

Condition: Root Canal

Primary treatment: 1-3 visits to the dentist

Recuperation after treatment: 3-10 days

Time to full recovery: Up to 30 days

Condition: Appendectomy

Primary treatment: 1 pre-op visit, 1-3 days in the hospital, 2-3 follow-up clinic visits

Recuperation after treatment: 1-4 weeks, depending on whether it was laparoscopic or open surgery

Time to full recovery: 4-6 weeks

Condition: Knee Replacement

Primary treatment: Multiple visits before deciding to do surgery, 2-5 days in the hospital, followed by outpatient follow-up and physical therapy.

Follow-up care after treatment: 6-8 weeks with ongoing physical therapy

Time to full recovery: 12-26 weeks

Condition: Lung Cancer

Primary treatment: Multiple visits before deciding on a treatment plan. Surgery may be followed by radiation, chemo or both. Frequently requires treatment more than once.

Follow-up care after treatment: 4 weeks to 24 months if remission occurs. Ongoing scans to confirm cancer-free status, every 3-12 months for 5 years.

Time to full recovery: 5 years with life-long awareness of being at above-average risk of cancer recurrence or above-average risk of developing another kind of cancer.

Condition: Addiction

<u>Primary treatment</u>: Multiple visits and/or treatment episodes before the patient genuinely invests in recovery. Then, 4-12 weeks of residential treatment, and/or 8-26 weeks of intensive outpatient (IOP) treatment followed by aftercare. Frequently requires treatment more than once.

<u>Recuperation period after treatment</u>: 13-24 months with ongoing aftercare.

<u>Time to full recovery</u>: 5 years with ongoing attention to sustaining recovery and life-long awareness of the risk for relapse or the risk for developing another addiction.

Formal Treatment vs. Self-Help

When a person knows he is sick, is willing to follow recommendations to learn about his condition and decides to become entirely willing to do whatever he has to do to get well, he might not even have to seek professional treatment. There is a small percentage of people who successfully choose recovery through community-based resources like Alcoholics Anonymous or other mutual support systems. Those who make that choice and fully immerse themselves can experience profound healing and change. They are the exception though, and most require some form of professional help.

You might ask, "Why would that work if it is indeed a disease?" That is a very logical question! The first and most important aspect of recovery from the disease of addiction is abstinence from all intoxicating substances. Those who can successfully abstain by utilizing self-help resources can, in fact, be successful but it's because of their willingness to follow directions from those experienced in recovery without argument, resistance, or debate.

Rarely are individuals – especially young ones – able to decide to stop using, sustain abstinence, and experience true healing of their relationships and sense of self without the help of others. The disease is just too powerful! Engaging professional help from the start is likely to yield better results, even if more than one round of treatment is required.

Now, I know what you're thinking. You want to be "one and done!" You are determined that your family is not going to be on the "rehab rollercoaster" or going through the "revolving door" process to get to recovery. You are willing to pick a good place, pay the bill, and expect the results. And if your son or daughter doesn't "get it," then they'll just have to figure it out on their own. Right?

Ironically, we wouldn't blame the cancer patient if they needed more than one round of chemo or radiation (unless they continued to smoke, and in that case, some people might blame them). We probably wouldn't even blame the doctor or the hospital either. But with addiction, we often blame the patient for not sustaining remission, and we sometimes blame the treatment center too. With both addiction and cancer though, it is in the patient's best interests (and their family's) to follow recommendations for both treatment and aftercare with the hope of getting long-term results.

In many, but not all cases, your son or daughter will be recommended for residential treatment. If your son or daughter has health insurance, the insurance company will likely argue that outpatient treatment should be tried first, just to see if less-costly treatment can be effective. Depending on your circumstances, your son or daughter may have no other choice but to try intensive outpatient treatment first just to get the benefit of insurance coverage.

If you elect to try intensive outpatient treatment first, we urge you to get assistance from an independent addiction specialist in your area. To verify their objectivity, politely ask them if they are retained, compensated, or otherwise benefit from making referrals to one treatment program over another. If so, move on to an ethical provider.

Truly independent specialists can help you know which programs are abstinence-based and committed to protecting the group setting by discharging or removing those who threaten the therapeutic environment by continuing to use drugs or alcohol. Anything less than a zero-tolerance policy in an outpatient setting is a set-up for your son or daughter to fail simply because of negative influences in the treatment setting.

Ask independent addiction specialists in your area for an objective thumbs-up or thumbs-down before committing to any outpatient program.

The same is true when considering residential programs. Fight the temptation to take recommendations from friends, family, others who have been to treatment, or your insurance company. Treatment programs can vary greatly! Since treatment is a massive investment in money, time, energy, and hope, you want a treatment program that is a good fit for your family's needs, preferences, and resources.

Resources You Can Research for Yourself

It is so tempting to believe that you can find anything you want on the internet these days. And you can! But think about the differences between a fleabag motel and a 5-star resort. Both could present you with a website with pretty pictures and content describing incredible accommodations and services. We rely on brand names like Marriott and Hilton to help us identify reliable destinations. Unfortunately, there are unscrupulous treatment providers who are willing to exploit families in pain. So websites are an unreliable way to vet or verify the quality of care available at a treatment center. In fact, treatment has become "big business." For-profit parent companies are routinely purchased by corporate entities such as Acadia, Elements, and the Foundations Recovery Network. The parent name does not necessarily equate to equivalent quality programs across the corporation. That means that we cannot assume that the "Marriott" in St. Louis is likely to be equivalent to the "Marriott" in Tucson.

Think back to the "old days" when we relied on travel agents instead of Orbitz and Expedia. While accreditation symbols and word-of-mouth recommendations are helpful, the stakes are too high when choosing a treatment program for your beloved son or daughter.

roughAddiction.com provides customized matching services to help parents narrow programs to research. Working from our treatment programs across the country, parent consultants cross-reference parents' answers to treatment questions to match families with a shorter list of high-quality programs that are consistent with the needs, preferences, and financial resources available. Although the original plan had been to provide parents a treatment center directory, program changes are simply too frequent and dramatic to consistently maintain such a directory.

PTA parent consultants provide parents information about the philosophy of care, treatment environment, details of therapeutic services, financial information (including actual costs of care), and editorial comments based on actual experiences with the programs. Instead of wandering blindly through internet websites that rarely offer financial details, or disclose some of the less desirable aspects of their programs, parents can get reliable information for a short list of programs to help them make a final selection.

Free information is available through the National Association of Addiction Treatment Providers and the National Association of Therapeutic Schools and Programs. NAATP and NATSAP both provide searchable directories to help the general public identify their member organizations. The SAMHSA website is searchable by location and offers more information about publicly-funded services and can be helpful if none of the programs included in the Parenting Through Addiction, NAATP, or NATSAP directories are accessible or affordable.

Ultimately, following directions is easier if you have confidence in the credibility of the professional giving those directions. Although Parenting Through Addiction does not provide counseling services, private consultation services, and customized treatment matching services are available.

SO, LET THE DRIVING LESSON BEGIN, BUT ONLY IN THE CLASSROOM!

As treatment begins, so does recovery. It all starts with learning in a safe environment, just like the classroom part of driver's ed. Thank goodness they aren't out on the open road just yet!

Driving Lessons

 For an Adult Child with Addiction: Alcohol and drug use starts off as fun but it begins to make changes in how your brain works over time. It doesn't make you a bad person that bad things happened because of your using. But it does mean that you need professional help to get well.

 For Parents: Begin the treatment and recovery journey with the knowledge that 3 days of detox or 28 days of treatment will not "fix" this disease. It's best to approach it like the beginning of a college experience. It's a big investment that can yield great opportunities for your child, but those opportunities will not be realized in a few days, weeks, or even months. Plan for aftercare from Day One.

Doing your own research to identify treatment options? Visit:

www.parentingthroughaddiction.com/TheBook

CHAPTER THREE

RESIDENTIAL TREATMENT IS LIKE THE CLASSROOM PART OF DRIVER'S EDUCATION

The process of learning to drive begins in the classroom. Every day, the instructor introduces new material to the students. New lectures often cover material such as:

- rules of the road
- what all the signs mean
- insurance
- licensure
- registration requirements
- and a few basics about maintaining a safe vehicle

It's usually boring, and students often don't pay very close attention. The basics seem obvious – just pay attention and don't crash. Sitting through hours in the classroom represents a rite of passage to be eligible for "in-car" instruction. But learning to drive is a process, not an event.

Similarly, residential treatment includes a lot of educational lectures, too.

Counselors and other members of the treatment team introduce new material for the patients. Although treatment includes other elements besides psycho-education, lectures represent 15-35% of the content of every treatment stay. Lecture topics may include:

- The Neurobiology of Addiction
- Understanding the Effects of Alcohol and Other Drugs on the Mind, Body, and Spirit
- Breaking Through Denial and Other Defenses
- Step One: Recognizing Unmanageability and Accepting Powerlessness
- Recognizing Cravings and How to Manage Them

...the list goes on and on.

And just like in driver's ed, those lectures can often seem boring, and patients usually don't pay very close attention. The basics seem relatively obvious... "just say no." Or maybe, they are hoping to hear some suggestion, like "just don't use too much and everything will be okay." Yes, learning to recover is a process, not an event, too. Psychoeducation is one part of the recovery process, just like lectures are one part of the process of learning to drive.

RESIDENTIAL TREATMENT BASICS

Safety

All treatment programs should ensure a safe environment and that any medical care needs are addressed. This includes security of the environment to prevent entry of drugs or alcohol and devices that could be used to arrange for delivery of drugs or alcohol to the premises. The particulars vary depending on whether treatment is provided in an inpatient, residential, Florida-model, Malibu-model, adventure-based or wilderness program.

Education

Counselors give psychoeducational lectures with valuable information. Ironically, the information is shared with patients whose brains are still fuzzy and whose interest is limited or absent altogether. So, lectures may be delivered several times in hopes that, with repetition, some ideas start to "click" and essential information can be retained. But that repetition can make the treatment experience sometimes feel redundant and annoying. It can also lead to the belief that continued stay is unnecessary.

Therapy

Patients get professional help processing and sorting through all the thoughts and emotions associated with being in treatment, facing the shame and guilt of all the things that happened due to using, and contemplating a life without using. It is a LOT to take in, frankly.

Therapy takes place mostly in groups – with some individual sessions. Therapy groups are always changing because new people are coming in, some are graduating, and others are gone with little explanation. It's hard to develop much trust, but the counselors do their best to create safe group environments for patients to reveal their deepest fears, their most painful unhealed wounds, and feelings of grief over losing their most reliable companion (even if that companion hurt them). That trusted companion, by the way, is alcohol or their favorite drug.

Your son or daughter literally must go through a process of grieving the loss of their best friend. You see, from their perspective, their primary drug became very reliable in keeping them company, serving as a solution to one or more serious problems, but ultimately turned on them like an abusive lover. Remember that "Breaking Up is Hard to Do!" The desire to prevent that break-up is so predictable, as is the desire to convince one's self that "it could be different next time. S/he won't do that to me again."

So yes, the therapy part of treatment is more complicated than you would think! It's not just dealing with the wreckage of the past. It's also about grieving the loss of identity and loss of your son or daughter's most reliable solution. It can leave your son or daughter asking, "Well now what am I supposed to do when I feel anxious/depressed/lonely/bored?"

Fellowship

This is best described as formal and informal opportunities to swap stories with fellow patients, to learn about the 12-steps or other paths to recovery, and to hear stories of experience, strength, and hope from those who have achieved lives that are happy, joyous, and free. These experiences happen over smoke breaks, meals, at the gym or on the trail, during travel times to off-site mutual support group meetings, at different kinds of mutual support meetings, and around the coffee pot or the campfire. It is through the experience of fellowship that patients begin to feel a part of something bigger than themselves. That may merely be a "tribe" of others in recovery, but more likely it will be the 12-step community.

As stories are shared and discussions happen organically, your son or daughter can begin to know that others have experienced, thought, felt, and had some of the same embarrassing, wonderful, terrifying, and ridiculous things happen in their lives. They start to see that they are not alone and begin to believe that they too can recover.

While most treatment programs embrace the culture, process, and traditions of 12-step recovery (Alcoholics Anonymous, etc.), some programs create an opportunity for exposure to other recovery support systems, like Celebrate Recovery, Refuge Recovery, SMART Recovery, Spirit Recovery, Life Ring, or Bible-based recovery self-help groups.

Regardless of the context of the mutual support group, fellowship is the goal.

OTHER VALUABLE ELEMENTS PROVIDED BY SOME TREATMENT PROGRAMS (BUT NOT ALL)

Family Education

A family education program may consist of workshops, experiential activities, and/or multi-family therapy groups where family members get a taste of the treatment experience. Family members sit through their own lectures and perhaps even therapy groups. You may meet with counselors and attend an Al-Anon Meeting.

Family members learn some of the same things patients are learning in treatment. In fact, your participation in the family program is your little micro-treatment experience. By completing it, you'll get a tiny taste of what your son or daughter is engaging in each day. Your stay will be much shorter, but it will give you perspective on their experience in treatment.

When your desire to bail out or decline the invitation to the family program comes up, keep in mind that you expect your son or daughter to put in about eighty-five hours a week for several weeks. You expect them to be fully engaged. You expect them to learn as much as they can so they can be successful after discharge. If the counselor recommends that you come to the family program, are you willing to hold yourself to the same standard? We hope so!

programs, weekly family conference calls are an opportunity for parents to learn from the counselor, and engage in facilitated discussion with your son/daughter in a virtual family therapy context, or a multi-family support group call.

Taking advantage of all those opportunities will help you learn right along with your daughter or son. But it's not likely you were ever required to show up at driver's ed, huh?

There is no substitute for participating in the family program where your son or daughter is in treatment. If there really is no way you can attend though, it is crucial that you do everything you can to learn the material, put in the work, determine what skills you need to learn, and engage in your own self-reflective study anyway.

Parenting Through Addiction offers a multi-lesson online course helping parents learn what to expect from sober living and aftercare providers and other essential information to help you respond in a healthy way as your son or daughter progresses in the first year of recovery. Get this and other resources by visiting:

www.parentingthroughaddiction.com/
TheBook

Attention to Co-Occurring Disorders

Recent research has revealed scientific support for a claim many with addiction have reported anecdotally for years: that using the primary drug helped them feel "normal."

Ultimately that changed, as loss of control resulted in major pain points, but the individual remembers the substance offered a solution to a specific problem. That problem is often related to mood, anxiety, insomnia, PTSD, or even more serious psychiatric symptoms such as hallucinations or paranoia. Effective collaboration with a recovery-friendly psychiatrist can be an essential element to the treatment experience, especially if alternative, safer solutions to the "identified problem" can be found.

Finding and arranging for follow-up care by a recovery-friendly psychiatrist is an essential element of discharge planning for those with co-occurring psychiatric conditions.

A "recovery friendly psychiatrist" can be defined as one who does not prescribe benzodiazepines, stimulants, sedatives, or opiates to those who self-identify as being in recovery.

Sober Fun

Sometimes family members are highly annoyed or even angry that those in treatment get to have fun. Getting to treatment happened as a result of a series of very poor decisions, loss of control, and serious consequences that affected themselves and those who love them. So why should they get to have fun? After all, this is not supposed to be vacation or camp!

But just like everything else that happens in treatment, sober fun is provided for a reason. It is essential that patients learn that it is possible to have fun without getting high or getting drunk.

It is essential that they actually experience that fun, just like it is imperative that they experience belonging through participating in fellowship activities. If you don't believe it, check out the incredible TedX Boulder talk ("Transcending Addiction and Redefining Recovery" with Jacki Hillios) about the mission behind Phoenix Multisport and what they've figured out about recovery!

https://youtu.be/gzpTWaXshfM

There's also a biological reason for sober fun activities. They help the brain "kick in" by creating a rush of adrenaline, endorphins, and dopamine. Sober fun reminds patients of fun, substance-free experiences from their past that they have forgotten. Sober fun is especially important for those under thirty years old, since having fun is the perfect antidote for boredom, which is one of the biggest threats to recovery for young people!

Life Skills

Although you might not consider it, life skills education can be a valuable part of treatment for those who are younger and/or those who have never developed any life skills. That doesn't mean, by the way, that no one ever tried to teach them life skills or that they have none at all. But it is true that drug use often interferes with a young person's willingness to be taught things like: doing their own laundry, setting up accounts, paying bills, cleaning, planning, shopping, preparing healthy food, creating a resume, applying for a job, completing a successful job interview, and other essential skills for daily living as an independent adult.

Some treatment programs use the need for these lessons to illustrate what patients missed when they were using and what they need to learn to truly live independently. Such services allow clients to learn practical things while in treatment, thus giving them another way to learn how to ask for help and add value to the treatment experience overall.

Spiritual Healing

Although not all programs make the spiritual aspects of addiction and recovery a priority, many do. Paths to spiritual healing are not necessarily religious in nature (although there are some distinctive Christian, Jewish, Hindu, Buddhist, and agnostic programs out there). Many focus on experiential opportunities through encounters with the majesty of nature, solo "Vision Quest" experiences, the study of spiritual literature, sweat lodge experiences, guided meditation, prayer, and/or step work related to Steps 2, 3, 5, 6, 7, and 11 of 12-step recovery.

If your son or daughter self-identifies as agnostic or atheist, this should be considered when choosing a treatment program. While the 12-step recovery culture strives to be non-doctrinal in its approach to spirituality and would definitely not consider AA to be a religious institution, others would argue otherwise. Because making a good match between the patient and the program is so important, be sure to inquire specifically by asking questions such as: "How does your program accommodate the beliefs and preferences of someone who self-identifies as an agnostic or atheist?" Their answer, even if delivered in "politically correct language," will likely include hints as to how open the program is to other viewpoints.

Structured Living

Perhaps one of the most critical elements of residential treatment is the development of a structured daily life.

Ultimately, it is the highly-structured environment that creates opportunities for healing and recovery to begin. Your son or daughter is invited to learn, reflect, feel, express, cry, yell, argue, and decide which parts of the program they are willing to embrace. And by design, they are doing that with others on the same journey.

The development of structured living is one of the key elements of any rehab program. For the entire time patients are in residential treatment, the structure of their daily activities is decided for them. The structure of their day often looks something like this:

6:30am	Wake up, make bed, shower, and dress for the day
7:00am	Morning Meditation with the group
7:30am	Breakfast and Medication Pick-up
8:15am	Yoga/Fitness
9:15am	Break
9:30am	Morning Lecture
10:30am	Break
10:45am	Group Therapy or Experiential Activity
12:00pm	Lunch
12:45pm	Individual Therapy or Therapeutic Homework
2:00pm	Afternoon Lecture
2:45pm	Break
3:00pm	Life Skills (activities and assignments about financial literacy, nutrition, laundry, cooking, etc.)
4:15pm	Step Work
5:30pm	Dinner and Leisure Time
7:00pm	Leave for community-based Recovery Support Meeting
7:45pm	Recovery Support pre-meeting fellowship
8:00pm	Recovery Support Meeting
9:00pm	Recovery Support post-meeting fellowship
9:20pm	Return to the treatment center
10:00pm	Medication Pick-up
10:30pm	Retire to rooms
11:30pm	Lights Out

Weekends are generally a little lighter and may include sober fun, more therapeutic experiential activities, time to read and nap, or time to visit with family members. But basically, there is a rigorous structure for every hour of the day.

There are no options for refusing to participate in activities, sleeping in, getting a "pass" because of not sleeping well, feeling unenthusiastic, or disliking a fellow patient. Healthy routines are strictly enforced. The opportunities for self-imposing a structure on one's daily life do not exist during primary residential treatment.

Driving Lessons

For an Adult Child with Addiction: Treatment isn't prison, even if some programs have lots of rules. The rules are there to keep you focused (which is hard for you to do these days) and to help you get as much as you can out of the experience. It may feel like a long time to be away, but in the grand scheme of your life, it is a very short time.

For Parents: The time in treatment and sober living is an important respite opportunity for you. There are many people attending to your child to make sure he or she is safe, but that won't last forever. This is a crucial opportunity to sleep without fear of "the phone call," reconnect with the rest of your family and friends and attend to things you postponed because you were hyper-focused. The time will be over before you know it.

For additional resources lists, worksheets, and courses, visit:

www.parentingthroughaddiction.com/ TheBook

CHAPTER FOUR

LEARNING IN THE CLASSROOM AND PREPARING FOR THE ROAD

Driver's ed students and residential treatment patients are all learning about what to do and how to do it. Both are required to sit through hours of lectures of valuable information that is pretty dry and boring in the classroom context, but they all know those hours of class are a requirement to get to move on to the next step. There is a HUGE difference between learning how to do something theoretically and learning how to do it by practicing.

And yet, year after year, we ask teens and even a few adults to sit through the classroom part of driver's ed before they get behind the wheel. We insist on the classroom instruction because we know that learning the laws, the signs, and the mechanics of driving is easier to do without all the distractions of actually being out on the road behind the wheel of a car.

Likewise, learning how to maintain a life in recovery starts in residential treatment where it is easier to learn about the disease of addiction, the language of recovery, perhaps beginning 12-step work, and experiencing a life that is free from alcohol or other drugs... without all the distractions of people, places, and things that remind them of using.

Now, here's the tricky part.

Most parents would not willingly support their teen completing the classroom part of driver's ed, then heading to the parking lot, getting behind the wheel of a car, and driving away with no practical experience. While many parents are eager for their teens to become more independent, able to get themselves to and from soccer practice, and to get out of the chauffeuring business, we know better. We know our teens need lots and lots of practice before driving entirely independently.

And yet every day, families celebrate the treatment center graduation of their son, daughter, spouse, sibling, or parent with full confidence that the graduate has learned what is needed to know to live a drug and alcohol-free life in recovery!

But make no mistake. A "crash" after treatment and a "total loss" accident after driver's ed could have equally tragic consequences.

Even in 12-step recovery, there is a recognition that "some are sicker than others." The more powerful the addiction, the more important the aftercare plan. For those who have developed an addiction to heroin, crack cocaine, or methamphetamines, or those who used drugs intravenously, the risks of a "crash" after treatment are not only higher but potentially deadly. That may sound melodramatic and an awful lot like scare tactics, and yet that has been this author's experience.

While we always have hope for recovery – that it is *never* too late – we also never lose sight of the power of the disease of addiction.

It is, after all, a formidable foe.

Preparing for Discharge
(Aka Behind-the-Wheel Driving with an Instructor)

So, it is with great confidence (*over*-confidence, we know) that the newly trained driver's education student slides in behind the wheel.

In many cases, they have had some experience already – on the family farm, with "the cool parent" on a back road or school parking lot, or on the unauthorized joy ride. But it's just not the same when "Joe Hard-Ass" is beside you, clipboard in hand!

The instructor is taking notes, determining whether the student can correctly execute the 3-point turns, on- and off-ramp transitions, and navigate a round-about. He or she is giving minute-by-minute reminders of hazards, dangers, and laws. If only recovery was as easy as a round-about!

And no kidding. The driver's ed "graduate" looks very similar to the treatment graduate. They have that paradoxical confidence born of inexperience. Many young adults just want to get done with the class so they can move on to the next step.

Similarly, many young adults just want to get the "pass" from their counselor that they completed the program to either:

- Satisfy mom and dad that s/he did what you asked

-or-

- Prove to themselves and others that they can and will stay clean! Sometimes the intention is real, but there is a naïve perception that recovery will be easy now that they have learned what to do.

We feel so uncertain when young people are admitted to treatment. So often they really are ambivalent about getting the help. But ambivalence, by its very definition, means there really is a part of them that recognizes the need for help. Thankfully, this is where the typical student driver differs from some young adult treatment patients.

Perhaps the nature of adolescence is naïve confidence. It's often been said that "Adolescents have to believe in themselves and have to believe they can conquer whatever the world throws at them. If they knew how scary and overwhelming the real world can be, they would never leave home!"

As they prepare for discharge, your son or daughter will need to collaborate with their counselor to make choices about aftercare.

Your most important job as their parent is to convey your intention to hold your child accountable for following the counselor's aftercare plan, and to communicate your budget and parameters to your child, the counselor, the aftercare planner, and your independent care coordinator (if you have one).

"What is a reasonable budget?" you ask? Well, just like treatment programs, the scope is broad. You'll learn more about financial terms for recovery residences and sober living programs later in the book.

Parameters, though, are really not something we can define for you. Parameters include everything from:

- *Sufficient distance from your home community* – In general, we would recommend against your son or daughter returning to your home community. Yes, we know that they can find trouble anywhere they look, but in your home community, old playmates will come looking for them when it is known that they are back in town. So the question should really be, "What distance is sufficient to limit your son or daughter's less-desirable "friends" from seeking them out?"

- *Historically dangerous communities* – This may be a college town or resort community where your son or daughter has many memories of heavy partying.

- *State-specific laws* – If cannabis or marijuana has been a big part of the addiction story, then you will need to consider your level of comfort with your son or daughter creating the foundation for their community-based recovery in a state that has legalized marijuana for recreational or even medical purposes.

- *Reasonable distance for you to visit* – Since your son or daughter will be encouraged to create a new life in the community where their aftercare is located, you'll want to consider the implications of visiting there. Just as you want the community to be far enough away from negative influences, you also want it to be close enough (or at least convenient enough) for you to visit regularly.

As tempting as it may be to address the aftercare process the same way you addressed the treatment process (in which you chose the treatment program), it's best to allow the treatment team to collaborate with your son or daughter to identify aftercare resources. When you release control over that step (while still defining budget and parameters) it reduces the likelihood of getting into a power struggle and increases the likelihood that your son or daughter can begin to take a sense of ownership of their own recovery.

If you are unable to contribute any additional funds to help cover the cost of aftercare, that needs to be communicated early in the treatment process so the counselor can take that into consideration when making aftercare recommendations.

Keep in mind that different treatment programs have different philosophies about aftercare, just like they have different approaches to treatment.

Aftercare Philosophies of Care

Depending on the treatment program's philosophy, there may be more or less emphasis placed on accessing professional resources when your son or daughter's counselor begins preparing them for discharge. For this discussion, we will recognize these different philosophies as:

- Traditional 12-Step
- 12-Step PLUS Sober Living
- Sober Living PLUS Community-based Recovery Support PLUS Clinical Support

Traditional 12-step Philosophy of Aftercare

Treatment programs that place immense emphasis on 12-step recovery programs like Alcoholics Anonymous or Narcotics Anonymous will emphasize the importance of attending 90 meetings in 90 days, getting a sponsor, and "working the steps."

Attending 90 AA/NA meetings in 90 days

That doesn't necessarily mean going to a meeting every single day, but for every day a meeting is not attended during the first 90 days, there would be an expectation to make two meetings on other days. The intention is to help the newly recovering person continue the practice of giving daily attention to their recovery.

While in treatment, that was likely the routine, and the counselor wants to prioritize it as the foundation for the aftercare plan. But make no mistake, there is no question the counselor intends for the newly recovering person to continue attending daily meetings long after the initial 90 days... but they are just emphasizing the first 90 to get your child off to a good start.

Getting a Sponsor

A sponsor in a 12-step fellowship is a mentor who will guide your son or daughter through a series of specific steps toward recovery. Much attention will have already been paid to the importance of choosing a sponsor, committing to being guided by that sponsor, and "surrendering" to follow directions given by that sponsor.

Typically, newly recovering persons are encouraged to choose a sponsor "who has what you want." That simply means that, if your son or daughter hears someone in an AA or NA meeting who is genuinely content (and your son or daughter's goal is to be happy in recovery), then that person might be a good fit. Or if your child wants to be calm and comfortable in their own skin, then a person who seems that way might be a great sponsor for them.

Working the Steps

There are literally twelve concepts that represent the 12 steps of Alcoholics Anonymous and all other 12-step programs. The pace, method, and tools for working the steps will be determined by the sponsor and could vary dramatically from person to person. Your job as a parent is to honor the sponsor/sponsee relationship and allow your daughter or son to share with you as much or as little about their experience of doing step work as they choose and/or as recommended by their sponsor. Keep in mind that, while making amends to others (like parents) is part of the 12 steps, the timing will be determined together with the sponsor. It will likely be many months, maybe years, and perhaps never that your son or daughter makes amends to you, even if they are abstaining and working a strong 12-step program.

Deliberately avoiding Old Playmates & Old Playgrounds and Finding New Friends in Recovery: Particularly for teens and young adults, the need to distance themselves from the people, places, and things associated with using alcohol or other drugs is essential. Newly recovering persons are encouraged to get phone numbers from those of the same gender who have more experience in recovery, and make contact with a few people each day to help develop new friends who understand recovery. By staying focused on creating a new life, it makes it a little easier to stay away from those who represent their old life in active addiction.

Although not all sober living homes rely solely on 12-Step Recovery recommendations, many use that basic model as the foundation. Assume that all of the following require and/or recommend those elements of a recovery program, but some add additional supports and services.

Twelve-Step PLUS Sober Living

In many cases, one of the best things that could happen for a person in early recovery is for them to make a new life in recovery elsewhere, at least for the first six to twelve months of early recovery. So, parents should anticipate that the counselor might recommend transitioning from primary residential treatment to some form of transitional living. Words to listen for include: sober living, transitional care, recovery residence, or even (old school language) halfway house.

By living in community with others who understand addiction and recovery, newly recovering people have a better chance of getting off to a good start. It is generally easier to discuss the challenges of abstinence from alcohol or other drugs with those who have been on the same journey. Residents also have some degree of accountability (without the baggage of old resentments, fears, and hurt feelings within the family) to work a program of recovery, abstain from alcohol or drugs, share household duties, and demonstrate personal responsibility.

Perhaps even more than within the treatment sector, sober living and recovery residences have different levels and quality of care. The next section includes descriptions and examples of these programs as well as information about finances.

Virtually all sober living environments have an expectation for abstinence, but in 12-step-specific homes, there is also an expectation of full engagement in 12-step recovery. Each home has its own structure, culture, rules and in many cases, supervision and monitoring.

Sober Living PLUS – Community-Based Recovery PLUS Clinical Support

If it is clear that your daughter or son still needs to continue in treatment (which is likely for the vast majority of those who complete 28-day programs), additional professional services may be recommended.

Typically, those services will be offered through a separate professional outpatient treatment program, but sometimes they are included in the price of sober living (especially with Level IV Extended Care programs).

Partial Hospitalization Programs (PHP) typically meet five days a week and operate through most of the day. They include lots of the same kind of care that was happening in the primary residential program such as group therapy, individual therapy, experiential therapy, and psychoeducational groups. PHP is considered an outpatient level of care, but sometimes residential programs bill insurance for partial hospitalization days if insurance benefits for residential care have been exhausted. Unless you are prepared to private-pay, it is important to check with insurance to determine how many of the allowable PHP days are still available to be pre-authorized before you agree to that level of aftercare.

Intensive Outpatient Programs (IOP) typically meet three to four days a week, for three to five hours a day. They too include a variety of psychoeducation and process groups and may or may not include individual therapy. These are the most affordable of the structured outpatient programs, but you should still check with insurance to determine whether the benefit will cover IOP.

Many times, programs will recommend that families simply private-pay for outpatient care because insurance reimbursement is such a hassle. While this is true, do keep in mind that some of those programs' daily rate for PHP or IOP could be equal to or even more costly than a residential program day.

And just like the aftercare plans we discussed, participation in 12-step or other mutual support group would be recommended in addition to the sober living and professional clinical support. Programs that recognize the value of professional services are more likely to recognize alternatives to 12-Step Recovery for mutual support such as Refuge Recovery, SMART Recovery, Celebrate Recovery, LifeRing, or Reformers Unanimous.

Understanding the Different Levels of Sober Living/Recovery Residence Homes

The National Alliance of Recovery Residences has affiliate partners in many (but not all) states. NARR developed standards of care for different levels of recovery residences in hopes of raising the quality of care nationally, holding participating homes accountable, and helping consumers and families understand the differences between very-low and very-high priced homes.

There are essentially four levels of sober living homes.

1. **Self-governing homes such as Oxford Houses**

   These homes have no staff, few rules, and residents hold each other accountable for remaining abstinent, working a recovery program, and paying their rent on time each week. These homes can be very, very good or very, very bad! They are appealing because they are the most affordable (often as little as $100/week), have few rules, minimal deposits, and no minimum length of stay.

   It is easy to find out which homes have vacancies from the Oxford House website (oxfordhouse.org/locate_houses), but finding out if the milieu of the home is a healthy one usually takes much more effort. It is reasonable to ask the counselor, "Who does the continuing care planning?" to make an effort to find out if the house under consideration is located in a safe neighborhood and has a good reputation in the local recovery community.

There are a few other self-governing homes around that are privately owned. These can be good resources though, so if the counselor recommends one, don't immediately discount them. On the other hand, there are sometimes conflicts of interests. The treatment industry is, unfortunately, full of opportunists and those who wish to "give back." Some are highly questionable, while others offer excellent value and perfectly acceptable accommodations.

We recommend that you inquire with a local independent addiction specialist to find out the reputation for quality of care before proceeding to a privately-owned sober home.

2. Monitored Homes

These homes generally offer some paid staff who have the responsibility of providing recovery support, monitoring for safety and collaborative relationships between residents, doing drug testing and periodic inspections to ensure that all residents are drug/alcohol-free, and enforcing rules and curfews. Many monitored homes do not have staff who live on-site. Staff are likely to be present during the day almost every day, available to residents in crisis 24/7, and may make unannounced night-time drop-by visits.

By comparison to self-governing homes, monitored homes have at least some paid staff, more rules, minimum lengths of stay (typically three to six months), and generally more services for residents.

Fees for monitored homes will definitely be higher than self-governing homes and will vary tremendously based on location, accommodations, the ratio of staff-to-residents, and whether or not food, transportation, gym memberships, or sober fun activities are provided. A quick review of the examples below will help illustrate the vast differences between monitored homes. Some are very modest and affordable, while others are more luxurious.

Examples of monitored homes include:

Caldwell House in Lenoir, North Carolina
http://thecaldwellhouse.com/index.html

The House of Extra-Measures in Houston, Texas
http://www.thehouseofextrameasures.com/

DAYA in Asheville, North Carolina
http://www.dayarecovery.com

St. Paul Sober Living in St. Paul, Minnesota
http://stpaulsoberliving.com/

LifeHouse Recovery in San Diego, California
http://www.lifehouserc.org/recovery-houses

The Frog Pad House for Women in Delray Beach, Florida
https://thefrogpaddelraybeach.com/

3. Supervised Homes

The next degree of structure, services, and accommodations is found with supervised homes. In general, it is essential to make sure that the bulk of the difference in fees for this level of care is based on an improved ratio of staff-to-resident, additional clinical, sober fun, or complementary services. While luxurious residences can help those in early recovery feel better about themselves, they can also fuel a sense of entitlement. The continuing care planner at your son or daughter's treatment center can help you judge the value of a higher-priced sober living setting. Ultimately, while you may not mind paying the higher price, it's important to make sure you're paying for more recovery-related services than just luxury accommodations.

Examples of Supervised Homes include:

Oak Tree Recovery Homes in Asheville, North Carolina
https://www.halfwayhouseasheville.com/

Purple, Inc. in Atlanta, Georgia
http://www.purpletreatment.com

Power House in Gonzales, Louisiana
http://www.powerhouseprograms.com

Hartman House in Delray Beach and Boynton Beach, Florida
http://thehartmanhouse.com/

Hope Homes in Atlanta, Charlotte & Nashville (Hope Homes starts residents at Level 3, then as they progress in recovery, transition them to a Level 2 home)
http://www.hopehomesrecovery.org

Broad Highway Recovery in Richmond, Virginia
http://www.broadhighwayrecovery.com

4. Extended Care Homes

This represents the highest level of sober living care. Frankly, these programs are more of a hybrid between sober living and residential treatment.

These homes may be an extension of a residential treatment program or independent. If they offer treatment services that are billable to insurance, counselors should be licensed as professional counselors, social workers, psychologists, or addiction specialists. Depending on the state, these homes may also require state licensure.

At this level of care, families should expect some food, transportation, and sober fun. Like the other levels, there can be vast differences between programs. Some are luxurious while others may be quite affordable (but merely offer a better staff-to-resident ratio and more services in a simpler environment). And then, of course, there is the matter of location and the amount of competition in the area.

Extended care programs often provide care over a period of 3–24 months and generally have different phases of care. As your son or daughter progresses through the phases, the level of supervision goes down, the level of independence goes up, and the price per month should go down as well. The initial phase may focus on getting established in the local recovery community and developing better life skills, while latter phases may emphasize balancing recovery with work, school, or volunteerism.

Examples of Extended Care Programs include:

Jaywalker Lodge in Carbondale, Colorado
http://www.jaywalkerlodge.com

Foundation House in Portland, Maine
https://www.foundationhouse.com

Green Hill Recovery in Raleigh, NC
https://www.greenhillrecovery.com

Turnbridge in New Haven, Connecticut
http://www.tpaddictiontreatment.com

In Balance in Tucson, Arizona
(In Balance starts most residents out at Level 4 – www.inbalanceliving.com – then as they progress in recovery, transitions them to Level 3 – www.inbalsoberliving.com)

Balance House near Salt Lake City, Utah
http://www.balancehouseut.com/

Encore in Arlington, Virginia
http://www.encorerecovery.com

Benchmark Transitions in various locations in Southern California
http://benchmarktransitions.com/extended-care-treatment-program/

Therapeutic Communities

Therapeutic communities are a more dramatic form of extended care and do not necessarily compare with the other programs described here, but they are important resources for all parents to recognize.

Therapeutic communities are highly structured and long-term (almost all require a minimum 12-month commitment, usually longer). They provide therapeutic employment as part of the program as well as food, housing, transportation, supervision and support. These organizations have businesses in which residents work to "earn their keep" in lieu of large fees. In fact, some have no fees at all after a small, very manageable admission fee.

Therapeutic Communities are great resources for those who have demonstrated a long pattern of relapse. They are not typically appropriate for those who are new to recovery. While they may sound appealing (especially to parents who value hard work as the solution to all ills), therapeutic communities are typically populated by those who have been through treatment (and often prison) many, many times. Often therapeutic communities are their only choice and resource.

Examples of Therapeutic Communities include:

TROSA in Durham, North Carolina
http://www.trosainc.org/program-services

Delancy Street Foundations with programs across the U.S.
http://www.delanceystreetfoundation.org/index.php

Salvation Army Programs across the U.S.
https://www.salvationarmyusa.org/usn/combat-addiction/

** These homes are identified for explanatory purposes only. Note that not all the above-referenced homes are recognized by the National Alliance of Recovery Residence affiliates as accredited homes. Programs change over time as staff, ownership, and policies change, so please perform due diligence in determining if a home is right for your son or daughter.

This is best accomplished with the help of an independent addiction specialist or through a service like Parenting Through Addiction. Customized Treatment and/or Aftercare Matching Services are a fee-based service offered by Parenting Through Addiction. Ultimately though, we encourage you to accept guidance from professionals while still evaluating programs for yourself.

A Parent's Role in Preparing for the Next Stage of the Learning Process

The most important reminder for parents preparing for their son or daughter to leave "the classroom" is to remember that you are not well-equipped or prepared to do the "behind the wheel instruction" of your son or daughter's recovery.

While you might have been willing to teach your children how to drive, it is unlikely that you would have been able to teach them how to fly an airplane. So perhaps it's best to use that metaphor instead. Would you be confident enough to teach your son or daughter how to fly an airplane? At the risk of sounding melodramatic, death really could happen if addiction progresses, so it's best to allow experienced "pilots" to give the instruction.

Even if you happen to be a person in your own recovery, your son or daughter really needs to learn to apply new recovery skills on their own. A recovering mom or dad would never consider sponsoring their own son, so coordinating aftercare would be even more inappropriate. But make no mistake, a parent's role in the decision-making process for aftercare is essential!

1. Your son or daughter's counselor will need your buy-in before proposing aftercare recommend-ations to your adult child. Make a point of telling

the counselor, "I want to support your very best aftercare recommendation that is within my budget and my parameters. Please be sure to let my son/daughter know that your recommendation is the only thing I will support." Unfortunately, your son or daughter may be overconfident or still ambivalent about recovery, so your endorsement of the counselor's aftercare recommendations is essential.

2. You set the budget. Aftercare is like a self-funded recovery insurance policy on the treatment experience. Health insurance will likely help with clinical support but will not usually pay for sober living. If insurance deductibles and out-of-pocket maximums have been paid, then insurance may pay 100% of in-network clinical services. But remember, even if the deductibles and out-of-pocket maximums for out-of-network services have been paid and the coverage is 100%, out-of-network providers can bill you the difference between the amount the insurance pays and the amount they charge for the service. In some cases, out-of-network outpatient services are equal to or above the daily residential rate! So, set your budget, communicate it to the counselor, and make sure to get confirmation of what insurance is expected to pay and what you will be billed.

3. You set the parameters of location. If your son or daughter has been recommended for sober

living, and there are sober living options within your budget, that's likely the best option. But it's important for you to communicate to the counselor which communities/states are off-limits. For example, if you know that your son or daughter has a history in a particular community, it's best that they not go to sober living there. Similarly, if your son or daughter has a history of leaving programs before completing them, it is probably best to avoid a sober living home close enough to old playmates who might be willing to facilitate a premature discharge.

4. You define what additional resources you will provide in aftercare, such as a vehicle, phone, spending money, etc. If you do not want to provide some or any of those, it is best for the counselor to choose a program where that is the norm and/or a restriction in the earlier levels of care. Some programs provide bicycles and/or bus passes for getting around town for the first few months. Similarly, some programs are all-inclusive to avoid the need for spending money so that your son or daughter can learn to live within a budget (perhaps for the first time).

Once you have communicated your intention to only support the counselor's aftercare recommendations (not simply what your son or daughter wants to do), set your budget, defined your parameters and additional resources you will provide, it's best to detach. If you have been working with an independent addiction specialist or with Parenting Through Addiction, you may want to ask them to vet any sober living and/or aftercare programs recommended by your counselor (just for a second opinion), but otherwise, fight the temptation to go down the "rabbit hole" of internet searching again. Allow the counselor to lead your son or daughter to responsibly choose and commit to an aftercare plan as their first big step toward owning their recovery.

Driving Lessons

 For an Adult Child with Addiction: Consider a place that you might like to live that is away from home but in a location where you might genuinely want to build a life. Choosing such a place for aftercare can make it much easier to avoid outreach efforts from drug dealers or old using friends, feel less triggered by your parents, and more likely to cultivate true relationships with others in recovery. Find where you'd like to bloom, and plant yourself there!

 For Parents: You can choose the best possible treatment resource but without a commitment to aftercare you could be throwing your money away. Remember, aftercare is the "behind the wheel practice with a professional instructor" to ensure that the lessons learned in the safety of the classroom are applied safely and consistently. Ideally that place is somewhat removed from your hometown, because that will reduce the chances of relapse. But remember that you can visit them in their new community with the appreciation that there is recovery support for them there.

To further understand the importance of collaborating with professionals for aftercare placement, visit:

www.parentingthroughaddiction.com/
TheBook

CHAPTER FIVE

PROFILES TO ILLUSTRATE

Sometimes it is just easier to conceptualize the application of these principles as they might relate to specific kinds of clients. So, for the purposes of illustration, we'll use the stories of Olivia, Eddie, Mick, Erica, Jason and Nicole to help.

Note that these are fictional characters to offer illustrations, but there are enough similarities with this disease that you may feel like we are describing your son or daughter. But not to worry. It's just a coincidence!

SONS & DAUGHTERS

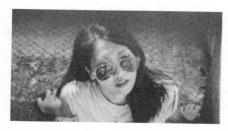 **Olivia** is a twenty-year-old who loves dogs, children, and video games. While always an outstanding student, she seemed to gravitate toward other students who didn't fit in with the norm. For many years, when other girls were experimenting with drugs and alcohol, Olivia was the one who would never consider it. She understood that

alcoholism ran in her father's family, and she just didn't want to take any chances.

But when she went to college, Olivia found herself feeling lonelier than ever. There weren't many girls like her at the school, and she never felt confident about boys. But her love of video games meant she found more in common with geeky boys at the school than with girls who were interested in sororities and pedicures.

In the spring of her freshman year, she found herself in a compromising position with some boys who had been smoking marijuana. She joined in, but was still apprehensive and cautious. She had smoked weed before, but not much. Over the next few months, they all started smoking more regularly and getting stronger strands from one of the states that had legalized marijuana.

One night, she was sexually assaulted by one of the guys' hometown friends. None of her close guy friends knew, and in fact, she believed that they might blame her for what happened, especially if she told the police. She had been wearing a short skirt that night, and she had smoked wax again (cannabis oil), something she had been doing more often. "It probably really was my fault," she thought.

From that point, Olivia began smoking more and more. She stopped going to class, began to have suicidal thoughts, and started cutting herself because, for some strange reason, the pain helped her feel better. When she failed all her classes for the semester, Olivia overdosed on her roommate's Ambien and Tylenol, and her parents were called to the hospital.

The psychiatrist at the hospital gave Olivia co-occurring diagnoses of Cannabis Use Disorder, Moderate; Major Depressive Disorder; Post-Traumatic Stress Disorder; and Other Specified Anxiety Disorders.

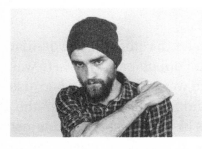

Eddie is a twenty-two-year-old guy who used to have the world by the tail. He was never a great student, but he was a natural musician, an excellent soccer player, and loved hanging out with his grandfather.

Eddie had always loved cars, probably because his grandfather did, too. One of his favorite things to do was help his grandfather work on his antique cars. Eddie was eager to learn to drive, and as soon as he was eligible, he completed Driver's Ed, suffered through the behind-the-wheel training with the instructor, and used money he had saved from summer jobs to buy his first car.

His use of substances started innocently enough with drinking a few beers with his friends, but he didn't like the taste. It wasn't long before he realized that weed was a lot easier to get, didn't taste bad, and wasn't detectable by his parents. Eddie grew to really like the way weed made him feel, but it was an accidental discovery that narcotics gave him energy that changed the trajectory of his life.

Eddie always struggled to wake up in the morning, and he was perpetually dashing in to beat the last bell, especially his senior year when he could drive himself. He found that he could sleep until fifteen minutes before the tardy bell, throw on some pants, and cut three minutes off his drive time by taking the back roads.

When Eddie had his wisdom teeth removed, the dentist gave him a prescription for an opiate painkiller. He was instructed not to take it if he would be driving because it might make him sleepy, and to switch to an over-the-counter analgesic as soon as his pain lessened. But just in case, the dentist gave him a ten-day prescription in the unfortunate event that he developed dry socket.

Almost immediately, Eddie realized that the pills did not make him sleepy. In fact, it was just the opposite! It gave him a nice little lift of energy, mood, and confidence. Eddie also discovered that if he popped a pill when his feet hit the floor in the morning, he was bright-eyed-and-bushy-tailed by the time he walked into his first-period class.

With the realization that the opiates offered a solution to one of his biggest problems, Eddie took all the pills from the dentist and found a buddy to get him more. The friend's grandmother had arthritis and lived with his family, so he always had access to a few pills. Over time, it took increasingly more to give Eddie the little lift he liked so much, so then he started snorting the crushed pills. Then when his grandfather died, the need for relief quickly escalated.

Eventually, he could no longer get the pills from his friend, and buying them was expensive. He had stopped working, never played soccer or his guitar anymore, and then a friend suggested he snort heroin instead: "Heroin is in the same class with those oxys you've been taking, and you can snort it. You don't have to shoot it! It's a whole lot cheaper, too."

By the time Eddie was offered treatment, he met almost all the diagnostic criteria for addiction, and he had been rescued from overdose twice.

Mick is a twenty-nine-year-old who works in sales for a major IT company. He started slow but seemed to really develop into a great salesman once he gained confidence.

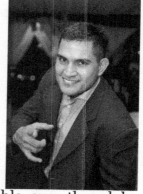

College fraternity life had given him the opportunity to experiment a lot. Weed, cocaine, and Adderall were so readily available, even though he had attended a rigorous university with a highly respected academic reputation. The culture had been one that really lived the expression, "Study hard. Party harder."

Part of developing confidence for Mick was getting over his anxiety when meeting new potential customers for the first time. Even though Mick no longer did illegal drugs, he had come to appreciate that his anxiety disorder was greatly relieved by the clonazepam his primary care doc prescribed, to be used only as needed. He had been just amazed that one little pill seemed to solve all that anxiety, and once that was gone, he was able to schmooze with the best of them! It didn't hurt that the nature of his business stressed the importance of entertaining clients with expensive lunches and dinners, often including alcohol.

Mick had not even realized that he was taking more and more of the clonazepam tablets, but he had noticed he was feeling worse in the mornings after a night of heavy drinking. He knew that his ability to focus and "stay on point" in sales team meetings was not as good when he was hungover, so he started trying to reduce his alcohol consumption.

Mick was surprised when he realized cutting back was harder than expected. There were even a few times he thought that he might be an alcoholic. But then he would rationalize it along these lines: "If I were really an alcoholic, then I'd be having the shakes or feeling some kind of withdrawals, but I'm not at all. So I must be okay. I just need to exercise more willpower."

When instructed to make an unexpected trip to Silicon Valley for a business trip, Mick quickly threw a few things in a bag and headed off to the airport. Once on board the plane, he realized he had left his pills at home. He knew it would mean he wouldn't enjoy his flight because he had nothing to calm his anxieties. Instead, Mick drank on the plane and ended up getting seriously drunk.

The morning hangover caused him to decide he just needed to stop drinking altogether, at least for a while. Over the course of the next few days, Mick began to feel worse and worse, and eventually experienced a seizure before returning home. The hospital doctor recognized that the clonazepam had been keeping alcohol withdrawal symptoms at bay and that Mick had developed a physiological dependency on the pills as well. Going without both had created a medical crisis as well as a wake-up call that willpower would not be enough.

Thirty-eight-year-old **Erica** is a highly successful real estate agent. Several years ago, she joined the ranks of the high-flyers in the local market, and now her name recognition results in a steady stream of new customers in the premium market every year.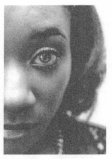

The daily routine of successful real estate brokers is highly flexible, and Erica enjoyed being able to create her own schedule, make adjustments when she wanted to, and never have to meet customers in the mornings.

Erica had known since high school that she could drink more than most of her friends, even the guys, so she never had any trouble maintaining her composure when she drank at after-hours functions in town. But she was cautious to make sure no one ever knew how much she was drinking in private. Her reputation meant too much to her, so Erica would never have been willing to admit that she needed help... because it might mean she would have to go away and leave her business.

Eventually family and her current boyfriend rallied together to stage a family intervention to express concern about her drinking. They shared their love, their fear, and their willingness to contact her broker-in-charge if she chose not to accept their offer for help. Thankfully, the interventionist was there to guide the family through preparing for the intervention, choosing treatment, and knowing more about the additional work they needed to do as a family.

Thirty-three-year-old **Jason** has really put his parents through the wringer. His early years of misbehavior as

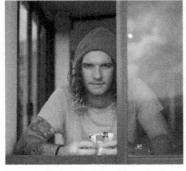

an elementary school student did little to prepare his parents for the challenges of the next twenty years.

Legal issues, suspensions, expulsions, traffic citations, "Minor in Possession" tickets, simple marijuana possession charges... the list just goes on and on. His parents rescued and rescued in hopes that he would "finally learn his lesson." His mother threatened to kick him out, but his father never could. They took turns being the "good cop" or "bad cop," but ultimately no one actually enforced any of the rules.

Jason's legal issues created an incentive for him to get into treatment, but he generally viewed treatment like a jail sentence. He would tell himself, "Tough it out until it is over, then get back to life as usual."

He went to programs that had funds for those who were court-ordered, and he thought everyone there had a similar story, attitude, and naiveté. No one seemed to recognize that the years were passing and that they weren't getting any younger. Ultimately Jason came to believe he was like Teflon – like nothing ever seemed to stick to him. He came and went from his parents' home, and jobs and relationships were short-lived and unsatisfying.

But late at night, when the party died down and the music stopped, Jason would reflect on his life. He didn't like what he saw. He had always assumed the time would come when he would give up the party life and decide to grow up. But with his legal history and his parents' discouragement, he had very few options. It was a sad life, and Jason became increasingly hopeless. The only thing that helped take away the pain was alcohol and more drugs. He knew his parents were there and still loved him, but his shame and guilt kept him from hanging around them very much.

Ironically, it was not Jason's criminal activity that helped him reach his "bottom." When he bumped into an old friend at a bar, one thing led to another. Before the night was over, a girl had died, Jason was questioned and released by the police, and in desperation, he called his dad to see if he could come home – just for the night. He was so tired.

Jason told his parents he could no longer live the life he'd been living. Jason knew he had failed to appreciate the help he had gotten in the past, but now he was really ready to get help. Jason now had the gift of desperation.

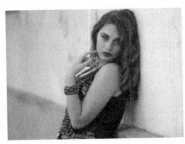

Thirty-five-year-old **Nicole** has very little family and virtually no money. She was never a heavy drinker, but she loved weed to relax after a hard day, and Adderall to give her the energy she needed to work two part-time jobs.

Nicole's mother had encouraged her for years to make changes and to stop using, but their relationship had been tense since Nicole became a teenager. They argued over everything: make-up, guys, school, birth control... just everything. She left home at seventeen and never came back.

In time, the reality of her life just got harder and harder to bear. She and her mother drifted apart, partially because her mother had a pretty hard life, too. Nicole had two young children, but her mom also had three other children.

One Saturday, when the boys were supposed to go with their dad, Nicole took some pills someone had given her at work. She had no idea they would knock her out so quickly. When the dad never showed up to get the boys, and she was asleep, the older son called his grandmother to tell her he was afraid. By the time Nicole's mom got to their apartment, both boys were sobbing and convinced their mother had died.

Driving Lessons

For an Adult Child with Addiction: It really is true that not all people with this disease are the same. It is important that your treatment program takes your needs and preferences into consideration. That means communicating what those are, so you have the best experience possible.

For Parents: Fight the temptation to let your insurance company make this decision for you. Even if you need to use in-network benefits, carefully choosing a treatment program that is a good fit for your child is one part of this process over which you do have control. Get help from an independent addiction specialist who has no affiliation with a program for the most objective support.

Chapter Six

Parent Profiles

The parents and families of Olivia, Eddie, Mick, Erica, Jason, and Nicole eventually came to recognize severe drug or alcohol problems their adult children were experiencing. For some, the journey was fast because they had no idea how dangerous things were, but for others, the writing had been on the wall for years.

Now their parents are charged with the task of identifying how to respond to their adult children's current crises. We'll use these profiles to help readers vicariously observe common parental behavior patterns.

Typical Parents respond with concern and commitment to getting their son or daughter the needed help. They don't know much about addiction/recovery treatment, but they try to take action to find help. The more they look, the more confused they feel because of the overwhelming number of options and all the scary reviews found on the internet about treatment programs. They are willing to take direction but feel like they ought to be smart enough to figure some things out for themselves.

Reactive Parents do just that – they react. They react with anger or panic by shaming/blaming/scolding their son or daughter for being stupid, irresponsible, and ungrateful. These parents show anger on the outside (and they really are angry), but they are also scared. Sometimes they are embarrassed because their image in the community is one they are proud of and have worked hard to establish. They hope that by laying down the law, their son or daughter will make changes out of fear now before things get worse later.

Naïve Parents dismiss professional recommendations and listen to their son or daughter. They tend to believe their child who reports: "It just happened the one time. That was literally the first time I've ever done drugs, and I know now that it'll be the last time, too." They may also recall their own youthful indiscretions and assume the problems at hand are no different from their own at that age. These parents are eager to show their son or daughter that they believe and trust them to make better decisions. They want their child to know they can learn from their mistakes (just like they did). While demonstrating trust, confidence, and hope are all positive parental qualities, these parents seem to be unable to recognize the seriousness of the present situation and take direction from professionals.

Bewildered Parents struggle to reconcile the difference between how they thought their son or daughter was functioning and the recent drug or alcohol-related crisis. As far as they knew, everything was going great... until it wasn't! They feel blindsided, confused, uncertain, and unprepared to take action because it all feels so new. These parents are not unwilling to take direction from professionals, but they are just in shock.

Equipped Parents get proactive when first learning their son or daughter's use of drugs or alcohol might be getting out of hand. They start learning what to look for, allow their son or daughter to experience consequences, and become ready to offer help when the time seems right. When a crisis presents itself, they listen to the doctors, make an effort to listen to their son or daughter (as much as is shared), and offer treatment. They don't believe they can personally get their child well, but they do strive to maintain a strong, loving relationship while hoping their son or daughter will accept treatment to begin to get well.

Waiting for the willingness for a son or daughter to accept help can be an exercise in patience, flexibility, and courage. The "hurry-up-and-wait" of taking proactive steps to be ready when the time comes is paired with the need to "sit tight" until that time. In that interim period, some parents find it helpful to arrange for weekly family dinners at a favorite restaurant as a way of staying in touch, making sure they get a good meal, and creating an easier opportunity for their son or daughter to say, "Yes, I think I'm ready." With that emergence of willingness, swift action is essential.

So, how can each set of parents choose to respond to the crisis at hand in ways that help them shift from typical, reactive, naïve, or bewildered parents to being equipped parents?

Let's explore the following opportunities for our profile families.

Olivia's parents quickly learn that an acute care hospital will provide primary medical care to make sure she stabilizes medically from her overdose. They may or may not transition her into a true psychiatric unit, depending on her willingness to stay and whether or not she is reporting suicidal thoughts. If she is not willing to stay and not reporting suicidal thinking, they will likely discharge Olivia as soon as she is medically stable.

Primary Treatment Decisions: Olivia's parents need to immediately engage the services of an independent addiction specialist, preferably before Olivia is discharged from the hospital. They need assistance to identify treatment options that consider all of the following:

- Diagnosis of Cannabis Use Disorder, Moderate
- No need for detox services
- Strong need for trauma recovery support
- Strong need for further assessment and treatment of symptoms of depression and anxiety
- Likely preference to be with those of her own age, and perhaps, just women

- Resources that are within the family's budget and, if needed, insurance resources

The independent addiction specialist can help them know how to present the opportunity for Olivia to go to treatment in a way that improves the likelihood that she will accept.

The specialist will also offer comfort to the parents and attention to their fear, anger, and confusion. Especially if Olivia declines the offer for treatment, her parents will need to start learning as much as they possibly can about addiction and recovery for college students. They will need to find a tribe of support for themselves, and begin reading and studying about addiction and recovery so they can feel more equipped. The specialist will help them have more patience with the process of waiting for Olivia to be ready and to know that until she is, there are definitely helpful things they can be doing.

They will learn that each crisis is an opportunity, so when crises happen, they will be equipped and prepared to offer help. They begin to get mentally prepared to consider that the next five years are going to turn out entirely different than expected.

There are unique challenges for college students and all young adults who need recovery that Olivia's parents need to appreciate. They also are reminded of things they already knew about adolescent and young adult development.

Aftercare Decisions: Once Olivia enters treatment, her parents will already be aware that because of Olivia's age, aftercare support will be crucial. With the help of their independent addiction specialist, Olivia's parents learn about sober living programs specifically for college students, collegiate recovery programs, alternative peer groups, Phoenix Multisport, Young People in Recovery gatherings, and chapters of Young People in AA.

Learning about such opportunities will help Olivia's parents feel hopeful for her future and confident that she can make friends with other young people in recovery after discharge. By choosing to become equipped with the help of an independent addiction specialist, Olivia's parents start with a short list of robust treatment programs that consider her needs, preferences, and their family's resources.

Eddie's parents will quickly learn that some programs approach opioid addiction with the hope of Medication Assisted Treatment (MAT) as the first line of defense against opioid use disorders. His experience with overdose will strengthen the argument that MAT is the way to go. They will learn about buprenorphine in its many forms and combinations, as well as the differences between buprenorphine and methadone. Physicians will explain how buprenorphine treatment will allow him to get treatment as an outpatient without the need to spend his days looking for drugs so he can avoid withdrawal. "That means he'll be able to really get back on track, get a job, and so on." And Eddie's parents feel better.

Then, Eddie's parents go home to do research on their own about this miracle drug called buprenorphine. They discover it is actually an opiate, too. They find out that lots of people think buprenorphine treatment is just exchanging one addiction for another, and that there is a lot of controversy about it. Politicians and doctors love it, but people in recovery despise it. So now Eddie's parents feel more confused than ever!

Primary Treatment Decisions: An independent addiction specialist can help Eddie and his parents determine whether or not buprenorphine treatment is right for him or whether he would be a better candidate for an abstinence-based program of recovery. They can explore treatment options that consider all of the following:

- Diagnosis of opioid use disorder, severe

- Recommendation for MAT but parental uncertainty about following those recommendations

- A preference to find a program that could give Eddie a chance to incorporate his love of music into his treatment experience

- Recognition of the possible need to address unresolved grief associated with the death of his grandfather

- Because Eddie is twenty-two, has no history of prior treatment, has no savings, and seems somewhat ambivalent about recovery, financial responsibility for treatment expenses could fall on his parents. Thankfully, he is still on their insurance. So Eddie's parents will need to decide whether or not to choose an in-network or out-of-network program. They will learn that sometimes out-of-network programs offer more creative, experiential opportunities to explore recovery, but their cash-out-of-pocket responsibility will be higher.

- If Eddie's parents allow insurance to pay more of the primary treatment expenses, then they can save their cash funds to apply toward sober living and aftercare expenses (some or all of which will not be covered by insurance).

Aftercare Decisions: Eddie's parents have no problem considering the likely need for him to relocate to a community in which he can make new friends and build a life where he is only known as a person in recovery. They are exhausted with worrying and ready to have a chance to refocus on their own lives. They also know Eddie's bad reputation is so well-known locally that he will need to establish a new identity elsewhere if he is to be successful.

One of the big decisions will be to gauge Eddie's degree of investment in his own recovery. The more invested he seems in treatment, the more likely it will be that investing in a long-term clinically supported aftercare program will be a wise one. But if not, they may need to hold onto their cash if they need to pay for treatment again down the road. But if Eddie really shows a significant shift in attitude, thinking, and behavior, then he could have a real chance to completely turn his life around in recovery. He will likely need some kind of psychiatric support, relapse prevention counseling, a recovery coach, perhaps even a job/life skills coach, and safe, recovery-friendly housing.

Mick's parents are likely feeling completely blindsided because they never really had any idea they needed to worry about addiction. There was no family history of addiction, only anxiety, and Mick's mom had been prescribed medications for years with no identified problems. When they learn that Mick is in the hospital, they feel completely unprepared.

Because Mick was away from home when he experienced the seizure, his parents will need to decide whether or not to go to him, wait for him to be discharged and then meet with him, or enlist the assistance of a sober companion, an independent addiction specialist, or interventionist. Frankly, Mick's denial is likely to return quickly after the shock of his seizure passes, so swift engagement will be especially critical.

Primary Treatment Decisions: In considering treatment options, it will be essential to determine if Mick would be a better candidate for intensive outpatient treatment or residential care. Some variables include:

- Diagnoses of Alcohol Use Disorder, Moderate and Sedative Use Disorder, Moderate

- Mick's desire to avoid disrupting his career by taking considerable time off work. Mick's employer has more than 50 employees, and he has been employed there more than one year. That means Mick is eligible for up to 12 weeks of medical leave without fear of losing his job (due to the Family Medical Leave Act – FMLA). FMLA requests must be completed by a physician, but the confidential information is strictly protected by Human Resources.

- Mick could take time off but might prefer to participate in treatment at night instead of interrupting his career. If Mick can embrace his need for treatment and recovery without a lot of denial, IOP might be appropriate.

- *But*, if Mick's denial returns or he seems more invested in protecting his career than engaging in treatment and recovery, a residential program may be necessary.

- A residential program that serves more mature, high-achievers might be a better fit for Mick, even though he is under thirty. For him to be in treatment with the eighteen to thirty-year-old underachieving crowd could be insulting and increase his denial if he starts comparing their often-stunted emotional, financial, and professional development to his own. Although employed in business (not law, medicine, or pharmacy), he may be best served in an environment that works with professionals since there will be a mix of younger and older accomplished professionals.

- While utilizing insurance could be important, it is more likely that an out-of-network provider may be necessary to accomplish the goal of helping Mick connect with other high-achievers in treatment. Since Mick has tended to be a steady producer, his parents might encourage him to take responsibility for some or all his treatment fees since he has resources to pay his own way.

Aftercare Decisions: Because Mick's job is a good one that has brought him a lot of pride and success, it will be important to explore ways to help him keep the job while prioritizing recovery. With FMLA, he can take as long as 12 weeks in medical leave without losing his job, but he will have a hard time agreeing to stay away from work for that long.

Mick's best opportunity for getting off to a good start in recovery would be to prioritize recovery for his first two weeks after treatment before returning to work. That way he can get started in an aftercare specific intensive outpatient program, get established with the local recovery community, and identify a few peers in recovery in his home community before returning to work.

Erica's parents, boyfriend, and girlfriends enlisted the services of a professional interventionist because none of them had been successful in their one-on-one efforts to talk with her about their worry. The interventionist set out a plan for them to follow and helped them choose a treatment program.

Primary Treatment Decisions: By working with the interventionist in advance, they were already prepared with a treatment center that considered:

- Diagnosis of Alcohol Use Disorder, Moderate

- The opportunity to engage in treatment only with other women because of her tendency to delight in the act of attracting the attention of men

- Her need to have some time to collaborate with her broker-in-charge to make plans to hand off her current listings to other agents

- Avoidance of being in treatment with potential clients and/or colleagues, since that was one of the things that kept her from going to AA meetings previously

- Exploration of her ambivalence about marriage, motherhood, and even whether she is in the right career

- A strong commitment to engaging the family in Erica's treatment and that will collaborate with the interventionist's approach to family recovery

- Identifies a community of professional women in recovery

Part of the interventionist's role was also to encourage Erica's parents and boyfriend to engage in their own recovery actively. They had tended to focus all their energies on what they needed to do to get Erica help, but they had little awareness of how much support they needed. The interventionist was deliberate in her encouragement for them to attend the family program at the treatment center, engage in Al-Anon, and to start looking at their own patterns of drinking. They were encouraged to get counseling to address their resentments toward Erica and each other. She was clear that after Erica admits to treatment, she expects the family to keep meeting with her regularly and that their future meetings include Erica after her discharge from treatment.

While Erica's parents and boyfriend are a little confused, they know their efforts to get Erica to make changes over the years have led to more and more arguments, secrets, lies, and manipulation by all of them. They know there really is a lot to do, and so they reluctantly agree to collaborate with Erica and the interventionist in a program of family recovery.

Aftercare Decisions: The degree of readiness Erica feels to return to work will likely play a significant role in determining aftercare plans. If Erica delves deep into her unresolved resentments and emotional wounds, she may need an extended period of time off of work. On the other hand, her need to return to the job sooner may be necessary for financial reasons. If Erica's boyfriend has done significant work to understand how he can support or sabotage her recovery, then it may be a supportive environment for her. On the other hand, if he has not seemed to grasp the role he has played in her addiction and could play in supporting her recovery, then it is likely she will need to move into an upscale, apartment-based sober living community with women peers in recovery. Family therapy, finding peers in recovery, and engaging in a long-term relapse prevention program will be essential for the first 1-2 years in recovery for Erica.

Jason's parents have little money left to help him by the time he is sincere in asking for help. They have spent so much money on lawyers, court costs, storage units, and living expenses for Jason over the years that they really do not have any funds to put toward treatment.

Fortunately though, a couple of years ago, they encountered a family education program that helped them get educated about addiction, stages of change, low-cost treatment options, and how to take care of themselves until Jason was really ready for help. They learned that, if things got bad enough, Jason might be willing to accept help if their timing was right. And they were deliberate about inviting him for dinner regularly just to keep the lines of communication open and to give him a chance to ask for help.

Primary Treatment Decisions: That night when Jason asked to come home, his parents were ready. They had considered:

- Diagnosis of Cannabis Use Disorder, Severe and Alcohol Use Disorder, Moderate

- The value of a therapeutic community that would provide a refresher course on the essential elements of recovery that Jason had already learned in treatment, give him a job and a place to live, and hold him accountable for working a recovery program

- They knew Jason would be able to enter for free but would eventually experience some satisfaction and dignity from working and earning his keep while progressing in his recovery.

- They took comfort in knowing that those who complete therapeutic communities tend to do very well. They develop new skills, a strong sense of accomplishment, commitment to recovery, belief in their ability to work and hold a job, and a belief that they now have a life worth living.

Aftercare Decisions: The most challenging part of the primary treatment plan for Jason and his parents is the length and restrictiveness of therapeutic communities. TC programs require a commitment of 18-24 months and allow very limited engagement with family and friends, especially for the first few months. It will be a hard commitment for Jason to make, and if he elects to leave the program early, Jason's parents will need to require him to provide his own sober housing and aftercare.

To improve the likelihood that Jason can commit to completing the program, they may explore ways to show support, stay engaged, and create an incentive for him to complete the program. For example, Jason's parents make a commitment to write him weekly until he is eligible for visitors. They will then visit at least once a month and make a point of learning as much as they can from him about the success stories of the TC graduates.

As a way of helping Jason prepare for his life after graduation (and to help incentivize him to graduate), Jason's parents agree to contribute money to a savings account for him so that he will have deposit money for an apartment after graduation. They recognized that they had been paying certain bills for Jason that would no longer be necessary so they would apply that same amount to the savings account. The caveat is that Jason is only eligible to get the funds when he graduates from the program and has gotten a job.

Nicole's mom had to get past her anger and resentment to be ready to help Nicole when the time came. Their relationship had been so rocky for so long, and she resented feeling that she had to take responsibility for Nicole's irresponsibility. She didn't want the grandchildren to suffer, yet she had struggled for months about whether to get involved to ensure the boys' safety. Even though she and Nicole disagreed, she knew Nicole made sure to meet the boys' basic needs, and she had no reason to believe they were abused or neglected in any way.

With the help of a counselor at a local non-profit, Nicole's mom and older sister had developed a plan of how and when to offer help to Nicole if things got bad enough. Her mom recognized how her pattern of shaming and scolding ultimately pushed Nicole away from her and might have even led Nicole to mother her own children the same way. She made a commitment to communicating differently, and it seemed that her conversations with Nicole did go better than before. Nicole's sister made a commitment to inviting the boys over to play with their cousins on weekends and helping them feel confident that there were other adults in their lives they could rely on and trust.

Primary Treatment Decisions: The counselor helped Nicole's mother and sister identify resources to meet Nicole's particular needs including:

- Diagnosis of Alcohol Use Disorder, Moderate; Cannabis Use Disorder, Moderate; Stimulant Use Disorder, Moderate; and Sedative Use Disorder, Unspecified

- Her likely desire for programs that were close enough for family visits on Sundays, that would allow supervised calls to children at bedtime every night, and that would allow her younger children to visit

- Counselors who are trained to help single mothers of young children work through their shame and guilt, explore solutions for working a recovery program while single parenting, and identify community resources to help make life easier.

- An age-appropriate education program to help Nicole's sons understand that their mother loves them dearly but that she had gotten sick and needed special help to get well. The program would give them a chance to meet other children who have had some of the same worries. They will hear from counselors that their parents can get well, and they will learn about some of the things their parents will need to do to stay well after they get out of treatment.

- Finding out from the local Department of Social Services (aka Child and Family Services) and from Legal Aid what could happen if a single mother voluntarily admits to treatment. Nicole is likely to be terrified that admitting to treatment could result in losing her children, so getting as many answers to these questions as possible can help.

- Deciding with the counselor and/or a family law attorney whether or not to engage the boys' father in the event of an emergency caused by drug or alcohol use. This can be a very wise or very risky decision, and is generally recommended that grandparents get professional guidance before making this decision.

Nicole's mom had done a lot of work to prepare for the crisis that she knew would inevitably come. So, when she arrived at the apartment, Nicole's mom knew that the time had come to implement her plan. She called 911 to get help for Nicole because she wasn't sure what drugs Nicole had taken, and she called her older daughter to pick up the boys. By arranging for them to stay with their aunt, they could play with their cousins and have a safe place to talk about what had happened with their mom.

Nicole's mom went to the hospital, heard reassuring words from the doctors, and waited for Nicole to come around. She explained to the doctor that she had been worried about drug use for years and hoped the present situation would create some new motivation to get help. When Nicole finally woke up, her mom was calm, comforting, and expressed gratitude that she was okay. Her mom explained what had happened and that the boys were safe. She was deliberate to avoid shaming, scolding language, and she waited for the doctor to explain to Nicole what had happened, how her body had reacted, and to offer recommendations.

The doctor was clear in saying that Nicole's respiration was so depressed when the EMTs arrived that she might have died had they not gotten to her in time. He shared the results of the toxicology screen and asked Nicole if she would consider a treatment program. Nicole was non-committal, but when she didn't adamantly refuse, Nicole's mom recognized that she had an opportunity.

Nicole's mom thanked the doctor and asked him to give them some time to talk. She then explained to Nicole that, while she suspected it wasn't the first time, the recent episode was clear and convincing evidence that Nicole had let her use of drugs interfere with protecting and taking care of her sons.

Nicole's mom explained that she had identified treatment program(s) that would allow Nicole to stay in close communication with the boys and help them understand what had happened. Nicole's mom explained that the program would help Nicole be the mom she knows she wants to be. Nicole's mom shared what she had learned about DSS/CFS and Legal Aid. She let Nicole know that getting help now could prevent her from being at risk of losing the kids, not the other way around.

While unpleasant, Nicole's mom was also equipped and prepared to say some hard things. She had practiced saying that she would be willing to report Nicole to DSS, encourage the boys' father to seek emergency custody, and/or seek emergency custody herself if Nicole chose not to accept the treatment offered to her. She explained calmly that she did not want to have to take such firm action, but she was not willing to run the risk that Nicole would not keep the boys safe. She also believed Nicole's desire to be a good mother could lead her to be willing to get help *if* doing so could help prevent her from losing custody of her sons.

Aftercare Decisions: Nicole may be a good candidate for a sober living home or Oxford House that welcomes both women and their children. Living together with other women in early recovery will strengthen Nicole's need to start allowing herself to trust others and ask for help. The more comprehensive programs even offer services for the children.

Nicole will need a recovery-safe environment in which to live, a strong connection with other women in recovery, and stable employment that allows her time to engage in both recovery and parenting.

After the first year, family counseling with her mother could be successful if Nicole is demonstrating responsibility and if her mother is more effective in supporting Nicole with less-judgmental, scolding communication.

Driving Lessons

 For an Adult Child with Addiction: There are books to help parents know how to parent through different stages of infancy, childhood, adolescence and even young adulthood. But there is no manual for parenting through addiction. Parents do the best they can and are strongly motivated by the desire to love you, teach you, and protect you.

For Parents: Good parenting doesn't prevent addiction, any more than bad parenting causes it. Be kind with yourself and recognize that this is just not a part of parenting you anticipated. You can learn to navigate through addiction and recovery as a family with the help of professionals, your tribes and eventually from your own child.

"Ginny and her team at *Parenting Through Addiction* gave our family hope again! They helped me learn the importance of being ready to act when my daughter finally accepted that she needed help.

—*Shannon B., Parent*

Chapter Seven

Support for Families

The support for these six families comes from several different resources and with somewhat different approaches. All of these resources provide help for families to become *Equipped Parents* who recognize as quickly as possible that:

- There ARE things they can do to prepare for a good response to an offer for treatment.

- There are some ways in which they are absolutely NOT in control.

- Becoming equipped with a good strategy, treatment options, and knowledge helps make it easier for their son or daughter to accept treatment.

- Being an *Equipped Parent* improves the likelihood that their son or daughter will not only accept primary treatment but hopefully those all-too-important aftercare recommendations.

These families found help through independent addiction specialists, a structured family interventionist, a local non-profit counseling center, DSS/CFS,

Legal Aid, an attorney, an emergency room doctor, health insurance, self-supporting therapeutic communities, and high-quality treatment programs funded through private insurance, self-pay, Medicaid, and non-profit treatment.

And most importantly, they discovered they could get help for themselves. The specialists they encountered helped them help their son or daughter access treatment when ready. They helped the parents learn, heal, and feel equipped to deal with crises until and after their child chose treatment. They also offered them a way to connect with other parents. The more connections they made with other parents, professionals, and the recovery community, the less alone they felt and the more confident they were in knowing how to respond (instead of react) to the person in their lives with addiction.

ParentingThroughAddiction.com is one resource available to parents everywhere. Members have online access to affordable, professional services to learn, connect, access resources, and get better prepared to help their sons and daughters.

The Network of Independent Interventionists, Love First, Structured Family Recovery, and ARISE are all resources to help parents connect to interventionists who apply a loving, respectful approach to help parents create interventions that lead to admissions and ongoing support.

Families can often get the names of independent interventionists and independent addiction specialists in your state of residency by calling the admissions departments of the state's best treatment centers. The treatment centers will only refer to those professionals with whom they have had good experiences, but independent addiction specialists do not receive any compensation or commission from the treatment centers. Sometimes talking with treatment centers is the best way to find them.

And lastly, your local United Way and local hospital can direct families to non-profit resources and publicly-funded resources in your community, region, and state.

Driving Lessons

 For an Adult Child with Addiction: Your parents love you more than anyone, but they do need help from others to help you learn how to recover. Their insistence for you to get professional help is not to suggest that you are the only one who needs help. Treatment programs and recovery are for the whole family.

 For Parents: Fight the temptation to conclude that your son or daughter is the only person affected by addiction. You have developed your own symptoms of all-or-nothing thinking, avoidance of conflict or discomfort, disregard for your own needs, and neglect of your other relationships. Make a commitment to yourself and to your child that you will keep learning, stay connected to a tribe of support, and begin to reflect on how you can recover through individual therapy, stepwork or family therapy.

For additional resource lists, worksheets and courses, visit:

www.parentingthroughaddiction.com/ TheBook

Chapter Eight

In Conclusion

Perhaps the most important message that we hope you get from this book is this:

*There is hope for recovery, and
parents can be a part of the solution.*

Because of long-time messages preaching Tough Love, "gotta let 'em hit bottom," and "there's nothing you can do until they want help for themselves," parents often feel great hopelessness and fear. Those feelings can result in broken marriages, parental depression and anxiety, parental self-medicating with alcohol or pills, and sons and daughters whose addiction gets worse before it gets better.

Your adult child's recovery works better when you let someone else give the driving lessons.

Driving lessons for you as a parent can come through a variety of sources. Sometimes it is tempting to assume that an author of a book is too busy or too far out of reach. But in this case, that is simply not true.

Through a monthly membership to Parenting Through Addiction, you can continue to learn from Ginny Mills and her team. You can view video lessons on topics such as:

- Balancing Boundaries with Compassion
- Balancing Expectations with Priorities
- Understanding Drug Test Billing
- Using Insurance for Treatment
- Understanding Medication-Assisted Treatment and more

There are also online courses to help parents know:

- How to determine if your child really has an addiction
- How to respond if you know your child has addiction but isn't ready for getting help
- How to respond to the challenges in the first two years of recovery

Members can participate in weekly education groups online that Ginny leads herself and have the opportunity for personalized assistance from her or one of the parent consultants that works with her.

To join Parenting Through Addiction for education and group services, go to:

https://www.parentingthroughaddiction.com/register /resource-and-community-membership/

To join Parenting Through Addiction for educational, group and personalized services, go to:

https://www.parentingthroughaddiction.com/register /consultation-and-community-membership/

We hope you have found hope for yourself and your family inside this book. We truly believe that whole families benefit from learning as much as possible about addiction and recovery. We also believe it's best to allow other professionals to help your son or daughter safely learn how to "drive" on their own, and it is best to insist the adult child take a gradual approach to independent "driving."

Lastly, we believe there is great relief for all when each member of the family can find their own tribe of support for recovery. It won't be easy, but it's easier with help.

Traveling mercies to you on your journey of parenting through addiction toward recovery.

About the Author

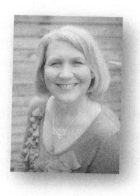

Ginny H. Mills is a licensed clinical addiction specialist and licensed professional counselor with over 30 years of experience in behavioral health. She holds undergraduate and graduate degrees from Wake Forest University and has lived most of her life in North Carolina.

In addition to extensive experience in "front-line" counseling with adolescents and adults, Ginny also served on the NC Substance Abuse Professional Practice Board, served as the Chief Clinical Officer for the Partnership for a Drug-Free NC, and served as the Program Manager for a residential addictions program at the former Wake Forest University Baptist Behavioral Health.

Ginny founded Full Life Counseling & Recovery in early 2009. She is proud to lead an incredible Full Life team that delivers a full-service outpatient program including assessments and treatment matching services, intensive outpatient, relapse prevention services for professionals, individual therapy, parent coaching, and a free, vibrant parent education and support program called Parent-to-Parent. Full Life previously operated a clinically-supported sober living program, Full Life Transitions.

Ginny leads a small team of interventionists following the Love First model developed by Jeff and Deborah Jay. Most recently, Ginny and her husband, John, founded ParentingThroughAddiction.com (aka The Other PTA), where Ginny serves as the lead parent consultant and supervisor. This essential online resource offers an affordable, accessible online way for parents to learn and prepare to parent through addiction toward recovery. Ginny is passionate about recovery and feels honored and privileged to walk the journey toward recovery with families and wants to extend that opportunity to families everywhere.

Parents everywhere are encouraged to join The Other PTA and/or contract for private parent consultation and support through the website:

www.ParentingThroughAddiction.com

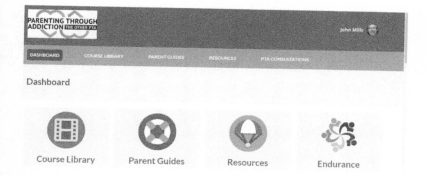

Made in the USA
Las Vegas, NV
27 November 2022

60466512R00080